Harper's BAZAAR

Fabulous
at Every
Age

Your Quick & Easy Guide to Fashion

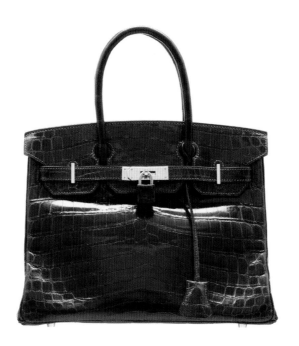

Harper's BAZAAR

Fabulous
at Every
Age

Your Quick & Easy Guide to Fashion

Nandini D'Souza

Edited by Jenny Barnett

HEARST BOOKS
A division of Sterling Publishing Co., Inc.

New York / London
www.sterlingpublishing.com

Contents

Foreword 6

 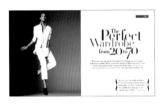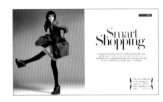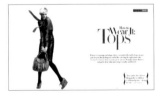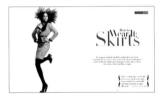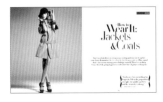

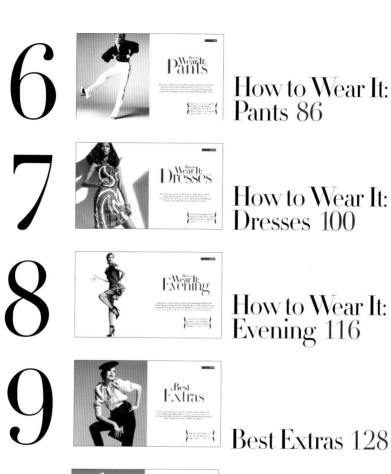

Foreword

I love spotting a chic, confident woman, whatever her fashion personality and age. It's always so inspiring to see how others put their look together. Even better is spying an especially smart-looking mother-daughter team—further proof that great style has nothing to do with the date on your driver's license.

That, after all, is what we're all about at *Harper's Bazaar*. We know that a fabulous wardrobe isn't defined by your stage of life—or your size or how much something cost. Looking great is about putting it all together with assurance and individuality, whether you're wearing couture or a bargain find.

With this in mind, we've put together this book, exploring the many secrets of dressing for where and who you are right now. It's full of suggestions and ideas: how to push the envelope in your experimental twenties; recognizing that what was perfect in your thirties may not work as well in your forties. And realizing that turning the big 4-0 (and 5-0 and 6-0, for that matter) offers a whole new world of sophisticated pieces that previously might have made you look like you were playing dress-up in mom's high heels. That said, there are also gems inside these pages that anyone can pull off.

We've found hundreds of looks that work across the decades and offered suggestions on how to wear everything from feminine blouses and basic white tees to a must-have pencil skirt and a statement bag. We've filled the pages with shopping secrets and best-dressed tips—plus picks that are great for every shape and the buys you'll love now and forever.

We also explore one of fashion's greatest hidden treasure troves—your own wardrobe. The legendary Coco Chanel once quipped, "Elegance does not consist of putting on a new dress." Never were wiser sartorial words uttered. It's just no longer practical to wear something only once before it gets shuffled into the back of your closet. Renew! Reuse! Recycle! It's a good motto to dress (and live) by. All it takes is a little smart styling that can transform what you already have into something fresh.

Bazaar is for you, the modern woman, the multitasker who juggles work, life, and a budget all while appearing effortlessly stylish, and this book is for helping you look as fabulous as you deserve.

Enjoy.

Glenda

Glenda Bailey
Editor in Chief
Harper's Bazaar

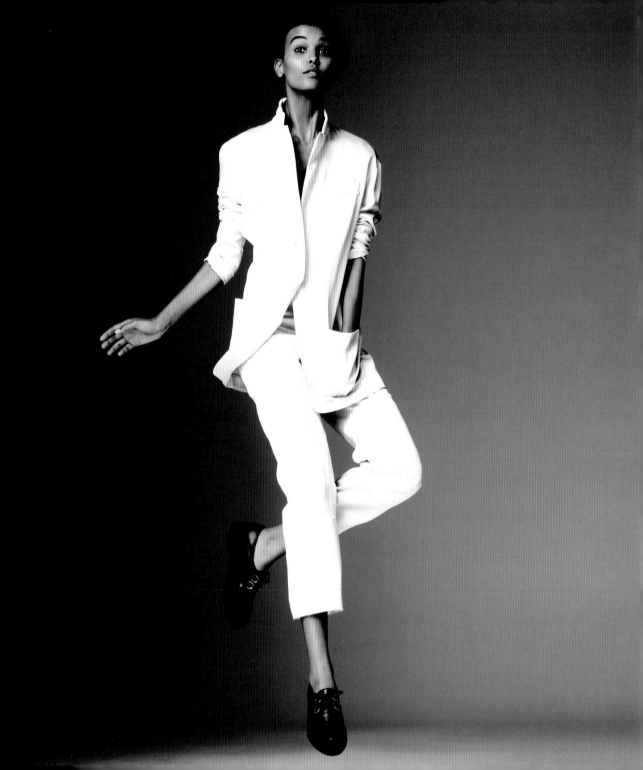

CHAPTER ONE

The Perfect Wardrobe from 20 to 70+

Whatever your age, great style is about developing your own unique fashion personality. There's no need to totally overhaul your closet every season (who's got the time or money for that?). Just pick key items that keep things interesting and chic, and make them work for you

{ "At every age, the ability to listen to your own instincts and to choose what makes you feel comfortable and confident is what gives you a great sense of style." —GIORGIO ARMANI }

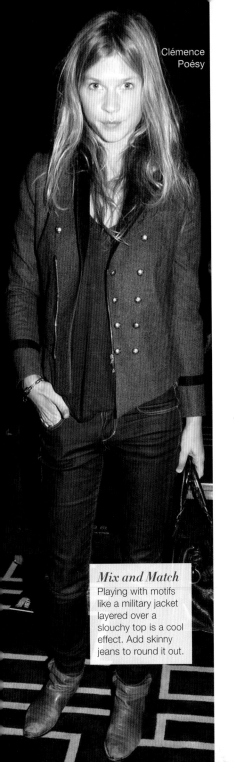

Clémence
Poésy

Mix and Match
Playing with motifs
like a military jacket
layered over a
slouchy top is a cool
effect. Add skinny
jeans to round it out.

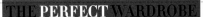

{ 20s }

This is the time to experiment and push the sartorial envelope in any way you want

Like a stylish chameleon, you can mix it up and play with trends. It's the perfect moment to explore who you are and have fun with fashion. You have the freedom to test-drive different styles without having to commit, and you can literally wear a different fashion cap every day of the week. Monday: Borrow a mannish blazer from the boys; try a hardware-festooned military jacket on Tuesday. Go ultra-short on Wednesday with a skirt as high as you dare, and dress down on Thursday in distressed jeans and a shredded logo tee. Friday, flirt with a sexy siren's dress. And then mix these all together with some great accessories for Saturday and Sunday. All you'll need to get started are a few staples: basic tees (you can never have enough), jeans tailored for your shape, a jacket, and a party dress or two. From there, take risks with edgier looks that express yourself. Shorts as evening wear? A peekaboo frock? A skirt suit dressed down with killer boots? Fabulous.

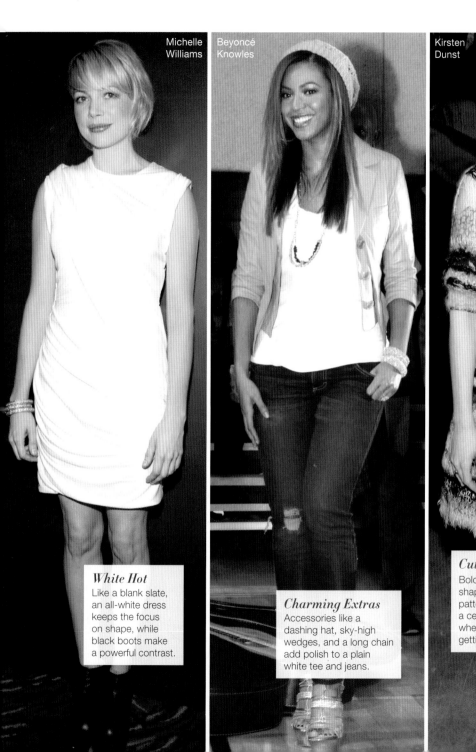

Michelle Williams

Beyoncé Knowles

White Hot
Like a blank slate, an all-white dress keeps the focus on shape, while black boots make a powerful contrast.

Charming Extras
Accessories like a dashing hat, sky-high wedges, and a long chain add polish to a plain white tee and jeans.

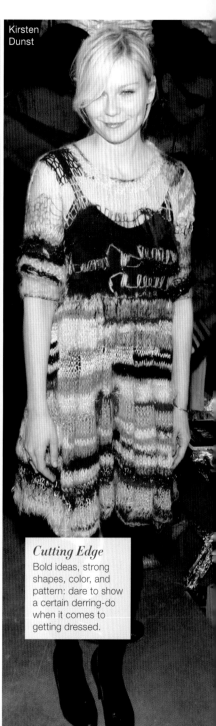

Kirsten Dunst

Cutting Edge
Bold ideas, strong shapes, color, and pattern: dare to show a certain derring-do when it comes to getting dressed.

Eva
Mendes

{ 3Os }

You've honed your personal style—
sophisticated but with a fashion-forward edge

So Sultry
When you pump
up the color for
evening, keep
accessories and
jewelry minimal.
A touch of black
adds drama to
vibrant red.

A few years in the workforce as well as in the social swirl and you've accumulated both deeper pockets and a busy schedule. Your daytime lineup is chock full of chic staples— charming blouses, a few pencil skirts, tailored trousers, and any number of great jackets. But increasingly you find you have to segue from day to night without having the benefit of zipping home to try on five outfits in front of the mirror. So how does one pull a plethora of looks from a bag Mary Poppins style? Make sure you have the right bag, for one. Buy a leather statement piece that can easily store a little sequined jacket or a pair of oh-so-sexy platform stilettos to spice up the tweed pencil skirt and filmy ladylike blouse you wore to the office. There should also be room for some wow accessories like bold necklaces, a gaggle of bangles, or a wide patent belt. (Likewise, there's also plenty of space to hide an emergency pair of ballerina flats.)

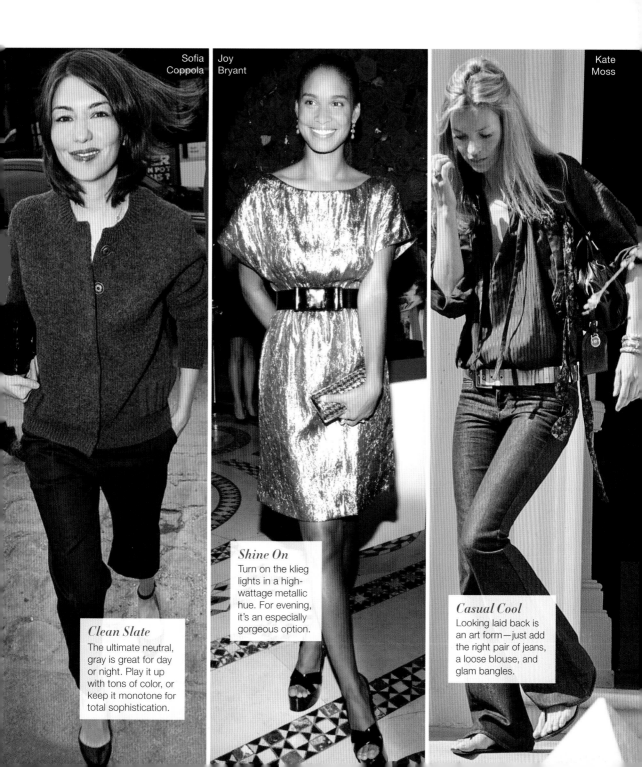

Sofia
Coppola

Joy
Bryant

Kate
Moss

Clean Slate
The ultimate neutral, gray is great for day or night. Play it up with tons of color, or keep it monotone for total sophistication.

Shine On
Turn on the klieg lights in a high-wattage metallic hue. For evening, it's an especially gorgeous option.

Casual Cool
Looking laid back is an art form—just add the right pair of jeans, a loose blouse, and glam bangles.

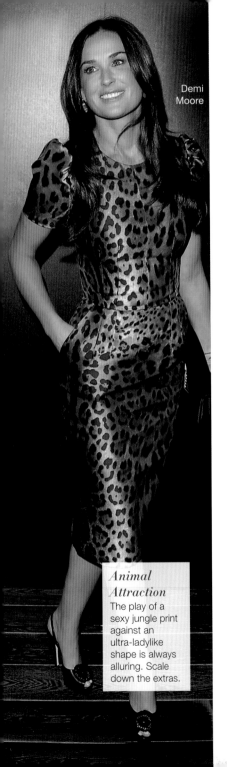

Demi
Moore

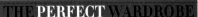

{ 40s }

You've found your stylish groove with
dramatic pieces that accent the classics

*Animal
Attraction*
The play of a
sexy jungle print
against an
ultra-ladylike
shape is always
alluring. Scale
down the extras.

Your mantra is polished and sexy, so swap out the minis for slim skirts and long, louche trousers that take your wardrobe in a more refined direction. Stick to the silhouettes that best complement your shape, and don't forget the power of a pop of color or how sexy a hint of shoulder, back, or leg can be. Sexy and polished, in fact, should be your motto now. Even if you live on the more urban, street-chic side of the fence, dressing is now about being pulled together. It all adds up to an effortlessness that comes from years of knowing what you're doing. An easy, pretty shirtdress is a knockout in a vibrant hue. For evening, you can pull off the more sultry looks that didn't necessarily look age-appropriate a decade ago. And as important as it is to buy only quality materials, it's equally wise to invest in a great tailor—someone who can make pants, skirts, blouses, jackets, and even a distressed pair of old jeans look like they were handcrafted specially for you.

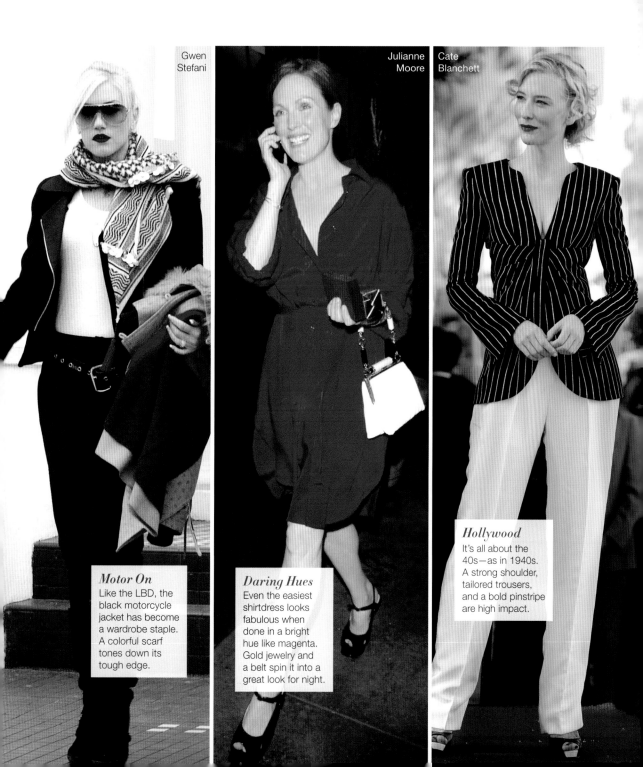

Gwen Stefani

Julianne Moore

Cate Blanchett

Motor On

Like the LBD, the black motorcycle jacket has become a wardrobe staple. A colorful scarf tones down its tough edge.

Daring Hues

Even the easiest shirtdress looks fabulous when done in a bright hue like magenta. Gold jewelry and a belt spin it into a great look for night.

Hollywood

It's all about the 40s—as in 1940s. A strong shoulder, tailored trousers, and a bold pinstripe are high impact.

Michelle Pfeiffer

{ 50s }

Confidence, perfect tailoring, and a subtle wow factor are a heady combination

In the Navy
There's nothing more stylish than opting for an evening look in blue. It complements so many skin tones and is ultra-sophisticated.

Fifty is nifty and the furthest thing from frumpy. All the rules—impeccable tailoring, fine fabrics, complementary colors—still apply, except now, being stylish has become second nature. You no longer spend hour after hour tinkering in your closet, cobbling together the right ensemble. You have amassed a terrific collection of the staples, plus singular odds and ends, that you know how to work into your everyday ensembles from time to time, and no matter the occasion, you understand instantly exactly what to wear and how to wear it. There is no second-guessing. Summer wedding after 6:00 PM? A clingy cocktail frock in a cheerful hue with some delicious baubles. Sunday brunch followed by window shopping? A loose coat nonchalantly thrown over a muted tunic and dressed up with an arty necklace. Swanky gala? Pull out *le smoking*. Weekend away? Striped shirt, white jeans, a handful of cashmere cardigans, and espadrille wedges. But you already knew that.

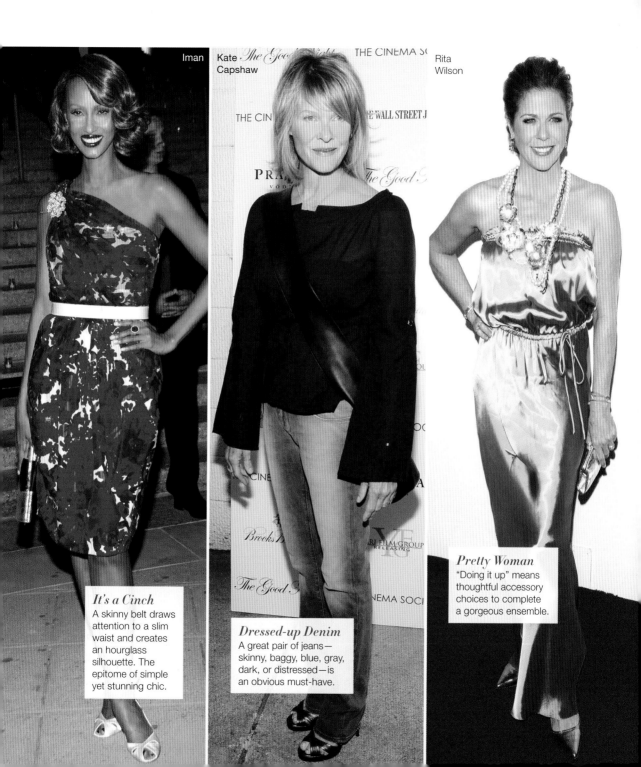

Iman

Kate
Capshaw

THE CINEMA SC

THE CIN   E WALL STREET J

Rita
Wilson

It's a Cinch
A skinny belt draws
attention to a slim
waist and creates
an hourglass
silhouette. The
epitome of simple
yet stunning chic.

Dressed-up Denim
A great pair of jeans—
skinny, baggy, blue, gray,
dark, or distressed—is
an obvious must-have.

Pretty Woman
"Doing it up" means
thoughtful accessory
choices to complete
a gorgeous ensemble.

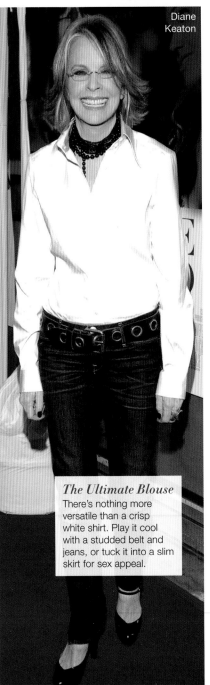

Diane von Furstenberg

Diane Keaton

{6os}

No matter the occasion or mood, you are the epitome of sophistication

You've cultivated your personal look but still have fun translating the trends subtly with a bag, scarf, or shoe. And you've got the fashionable gravitas to pull off something truly dramatic, like piling on prints or jewelry. One ensemble can be transformed umpteen different ways with brilliant accessory choices, like a pile of chains, a louche scarf, a metallic belt, or a necklace that draws the eyes to a delicate neckline.

Pleasing Prints
When picking an eye-catching print, like an ikat-meets-leopard look, make sure it's in a more muted color.

The Ultimate Blouse
There's nothing more versatile than a crisp white shirt. Play it cool with a studded belt and jeans, or tuck it into a slim skirt for sex appeal.

{70+}

Vintage or cutting-edge, classic or bold— you've got it all

The most stylishly forward women have a veritable treasure trove to choose from—chic suits, elegant evening gowns, the perfect pair of worn jeans, and any number of terrific layering sweaters and tops. Likewise, your collection of accessories and jewelry is a what's what of iconic pieces that have withstood the whims of fashion and are varied enough to suit every situation. No matter what you wear, you never look dated. And the best part? Pieces smartly bought decades ago still look phenomenal.

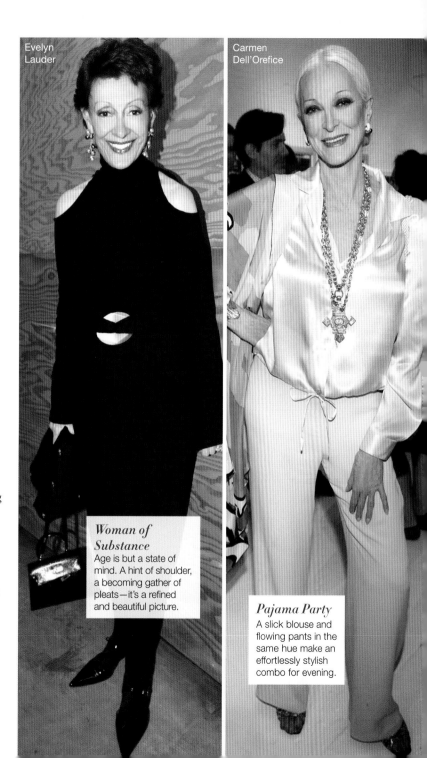

Evelyn Lauder

Carmen Dell'Orefice

Woman of Substance
Age is but a state of mind. A hint of shoulder, a becoming gather of pleats—it's a refined and beautiful picture.

Pajama Party
A slick blouse and flowing pants in the same hue make an effortlessly stylish combo for evening.

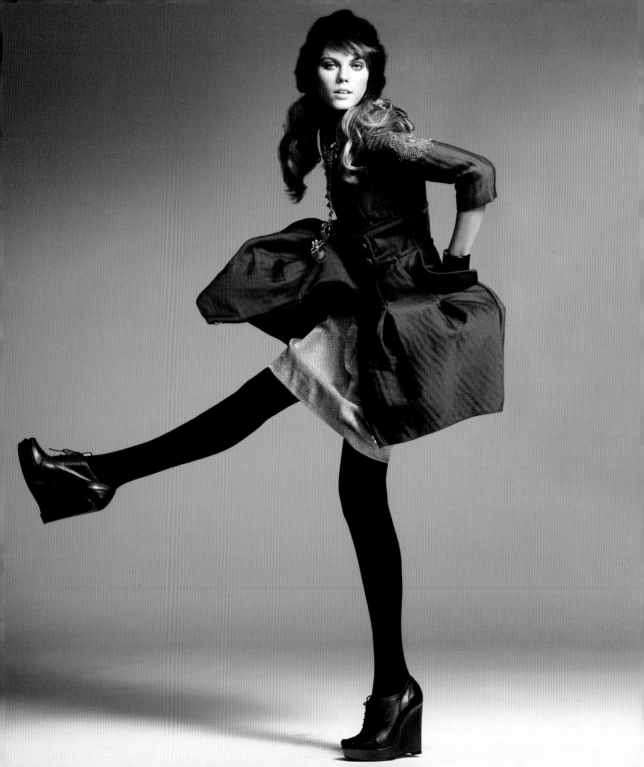

CHAPTER TWO

Smart Shopping

Creating a well-stocked closet is an art form. It's about knowing how to balance what you want with what you actually need (and already have), spending strategically, and recognizing what works for you: your lifestyle, personality, figure—and budget

{ "I like to mix high and low by pairing pure cashmere with a T-shirt, or flip-flops with a dress." —VERA WANG }

Know Your Shape & Style

Find the Perfect Fit

The secret to looking great is choosing clothes that look like they were designed around your body

• **To thine own self be true.** Before you even enter a store, know yourself. What cuts and silhouettes accentuate your figure? What colors complement your skin tone? What looks will you really wear (and not let hang in the closet for months)?

• **Every trend isn't for every woman.** Once you know what cuts look good on you, stick with them. If high waists don't flatter your figure, don't buy them, even if they're everywhere on the runways. There are enough great new clothes every season for everyone.

• **No two bodies are created equal.** Remember that what looks great on someone else

might not necessarily work for you—and vice versa.

• **Tailoring is tops.** Getting something altered, hemmed, or nipped in here and there can transform an item from simply good to absolutely perfect. It's worth it even for your jeans.

• **You can be in great financial shape, too.** If your clothes fit, you're going to wear them more often. Likewise, when you can look at something hanging on a rack and know immediately whether it's the right silhouette for you, you're less likely to make an impulse buy—which, as we all have experienced at some point, can lead to retail regret later on.

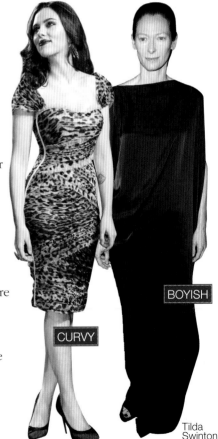

BOYISH

CURVY

Scarlett
Johansson

Tilda
Swinton

Cultivate Your Look

You have particular tastes in music, books, and movies—why not fashion, too? Develop your own distinct brand of chic

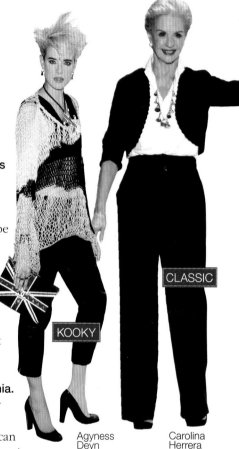

CLASSIC

KOOKY

Agyness
Deyn

Carolina
Herrera

• **Style setters understand the value of a uniform.** No, not a tartan pinafore and knee-high socks. The chic set follow fixed guidelines every day and night. Some dress up the basics: tailored trousers and cashmere sweaters topped with terrific accessories. Others always wear a particular silhouette but switch up the pattern and print to keep things interesting.

If You're...

• **Curvy,** go for fitted—not tight—cuts to show off your hourglass shape.

• **Boyish,** play with voluminous skirts and draped dresses.

• **Tall,** balance your torso with longer tops and low-waisted bottoms.

• **Petite,** don long, straight trousers or minis to elongate your legs.

• **Fuller Figured,** stick to structural looks that define your waistline.

• **A complementary closet is a stylish closet.** Once you've found your fashion groove it's likely that everything in your wardrobe will work together, and you'll discover more ways of creating great new ensembles. Even if you've owned a certain dress for years, switching up how you style it gives it new life.

• **Avoid stylish schizophrenia.** We're all for exploring new looks, but if you do it too often or too disparately, it can seem like you don't have a point of view. To that end, if you usually go for sleek, Jil Sander–like minimalism, suddenly trying to channel Talitha Getty might be jarring. There are subtler ways of working the look—try a few bangles, a scarf, or a pair of sandals (but not all at once) to achieve that free-spirited élan.

• **Don't force it.** If something doesn't feel right, like wearing webby knits when you're more of a sweater set girl, don't do it. You won't feel comfortable, and it will show.

• **Self-awareness equals confidence.** Wearing clothes that look like they were made especially for you (with the correct shape, style, and tailoring) will give you a major ego boost. And in the end, looking good is all about confidence.

Shop Your Closet

Your own wardrobe can be the best (and certainly most budget-friendly) boutique around—just check out your own shelves

Nowhere does the old adage "what goes around, comes around" ring truer than with fashion. Eventually, every trend, micro-trend, shoe or bag craze, and silhouette resurfaces. Sportswear from the 1940s and 1970s is ever-present, and like clock-work, 1990s-style minimalism reemerges hot on the heels of an especially embellished, overtly girly moment. Even Elizabethan collars have made a comeback from time to time. The savvy shopper understands this circle of fashionable life and will save the right pieces for the right moment.

All it takes is a little bit of imagination and a lot of organi-zation. Half the time, we don't even know what we have in our closets. Got a pile of V-necked sweaters you've been accruing since college? Save the ones that fit your style and shape, and donate the rest. That boyfriend's cardigan you've had just as long can be belted or pinned over a sweet dress or worn loose and baggy over jeans. And with the help of a talented tailor, you can pull off some of the more demonstrative trends. So what if you didn't keep your pegged pants from 1989? Take your trousers to the tailor and ask him to work his magic. And if you don't want to commit to the thread and needle, just cuff 'em and go.

Your accessories can be a trickier affair. These goodies often scream a certain season or year if you wear them exactly as you did in round one. Rummage through your jewelry box for the chandelier earrings you thought you'd never use again—it's time. But now, style them unexpectedly—to glam up a more laid-back ensemble, perhaps. A handful of delicate necklaces can be bunched and reworked as one chunky piece. Bags, especially, can look dated, but even these can be reborn with an artfully tied scarf or some new hardware. Try switching up how and when you use them, too. For instance, a teeny-tiny jewel-toned clutch can easily masquerade as a cool new daytime wallet.

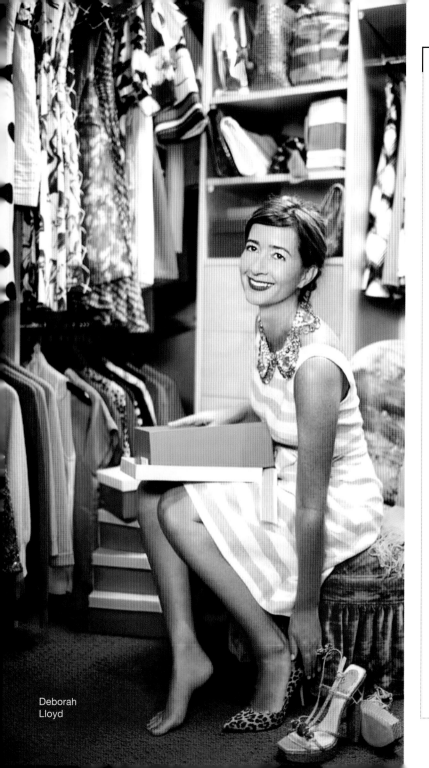

Deborah Lloyd

6 Ways to Organize

1 Start with the right hangers. Swap unwieldy options for slender fabric-covered ones that grip silkier fare and allow you to maximize even the smallest wardrobe.

2 Add one, subtract one. For every new item you add to your closet, try to take one out. If you don't, you will soon outgrow your space.

3 Seal in the chic. Storing off-season clothes in vacuum packs gives you more space for current goodies. It also keeps out unwanted pests.

4 Pouch it. Keep bags and shoes safe in their dust bags. You'll know exactly what's inside by the logo, and you'll also be able to hang them if you run out of shelf space.

5 Double up. Most closets don't utilize the precious space at the top and bottom. Reposition two rods so you have double the storage, maximizing floor-to-ceiling footage.

6 Separate church and state. Put your pants with pants, tops with tops, and so on. By grouping like pieces together, you're less likely to lose something—a filmy blouse won't get swallowed by a gaggle of skirts. And when you look at your closet as a whole, you'll be able to easily identify what's what and where it is.

Maximize Your Fashion Budget

Got high-end taste but low on cash? No worries. Just adopt these wise buying strategies

Mix High and Low

• **Wearing different price points is a badge of true style.** Any fashion maverick will tell you that the secret to great dressing today is in the melding of designer and not-so-designer. A lace Prada skirt topped with a Hanes white tee? Ultra-chic. It works best when you can't tell which is the high-end piece and which isn't.

• **Cheap chic satisfies even the biggest cravings.** Anchoring your wardrobe with one or two big-ticket items and then filling it in with more frugal purchases is a great way to keep on top of the style pile without hitting the bottom of the financial barrel. Disposable (read: über-cheap)

fashion is also an easy, guilt-free way to indulge in a trend you don't want to commit to.

• **Head-to-toe is a no-no.** Wearing just one designer is very gauche. After all, it doesn't take much know-how to wear something straight off the mannequin. The real test of "style-manship" is how different looks and labels are put together.

• **Even designers are doing it.** Every season, more major names dip their pinking shears into the mass market. Scouring these collections is a great way to get a designer aesthetic at bargain-basement prices.

Shopping Alternatives

There's more to scoring a great find than hitting brick-and-mortar stores. Here's how to stretch your fashion bucks even further:

• **Like Tupperware parties, but with clothes.** Host your friends at a stylish swap meet and ask them to bring along gently used pieces that they no longer wear.

• **You rent movies, so why not bags?** Web sites like bagborroworsteal.com, frombagstoriches.com, and borrowedbling.com loan of-the-moment bags and jewelry.

• **Gowns you can feel good about returning.** You can also borrow the current season's dresses. Stores like New York City's Wardrobe are cropping up everywhere. They take the guilt out of handing over cash for a frock you know you'll only wear once.

• **A season old but still as good.** Trolling the Internet still reaps rewards if you visit reputable bargain sites like Yoox.com and Bluefly.com. Be sure to check out your favorite department store's online sales, too.

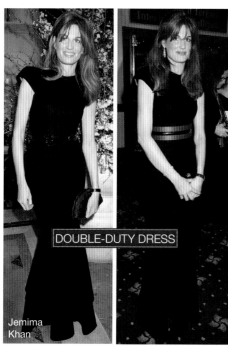

DOUBLE-DUTY DRESS

Jemima Khan

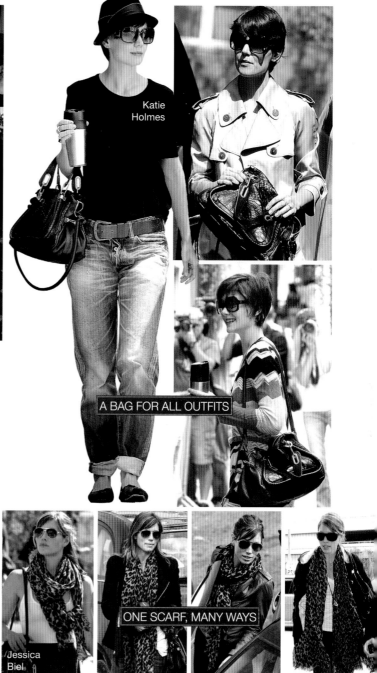

Katie Holmes

A BAG FOR ALL OUTFITS

ONE SCARF, MANY WAYS

Jessica Biel

Cost Per Wear: Do Your Fashion Math

The days of never being seen in the same thing twice are long gone. Even celebrities and socialites are recycling looks—including gowns. And every time they pull a dress, bag, or scarf from their closet, its cost per wear goes down. Even if math wasn't your strongest suit, it's a simple equation. Divide the original price by the number of times you plan to wear an item—daily, monthly, biannually. If the final figure is close to what you can live with, it's a good purchase. Put simply, if you're going to plop down some serious money, it should be for a piece you're going to wear again and again.

Buys You'll Love Forever

These style setters know that there's no better investment than a classic piece that will last a lifetime

LITTLE BLACK DRESS

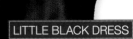

Holly Golightly lives on in the unmistakable sophistication of the LBD.

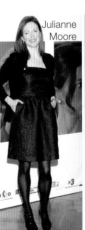

Helen Mirren

Sienna Miller

Its shape is unmistakable: a long, thin, elegant heel, a platform that gently curves in, a subtle square toe. To say that Yves Saint Laurent's Tribute has been a hit among the chic set is an understatement. In its many incarnations, it's the eye-catching punctuation mark to any ensemble, from jeans to vintage couture.

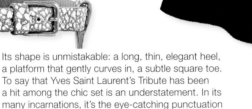

STATUS SHOE

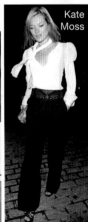

Julianne Moore

Kate Moss

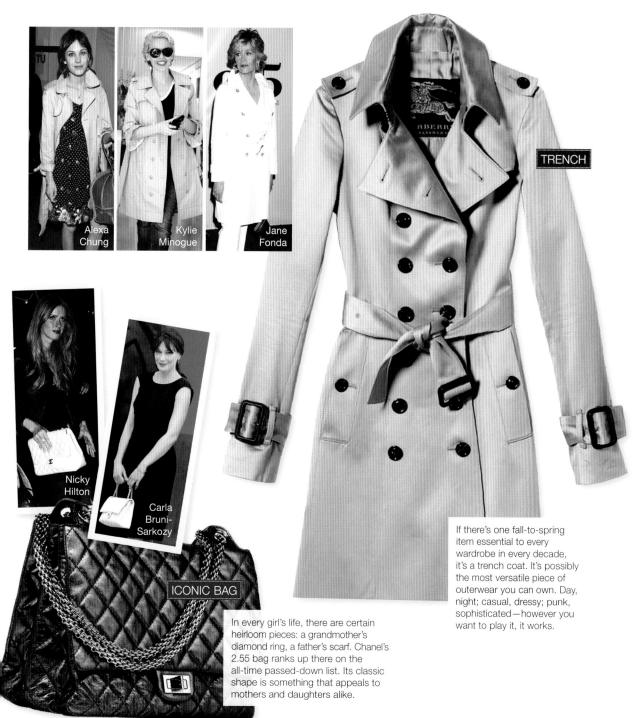

Alexa
Chung

Kylie
Minogue

Jane
Fonda

Nicky
Hilton

Carla
Bruni-
Sarkozy

TRENCH

ICONIC BAG

In every girl's life, there are certain heirloom pieces: a grandmother's diamond ring, a father's scarf. Chanel's 2.55 bag ranks up there on the all-time passed-down list. Its classic shape is something that appeals to mothers and daughters alike.

If there's one fall-to-spring item essential to every wardrobe in every decade, it's a trench coat. It's possibly the most versatile piece of outerwear you can own. Day, night; casual, dressy; punk, sophisticated—however you want to play it, it works.

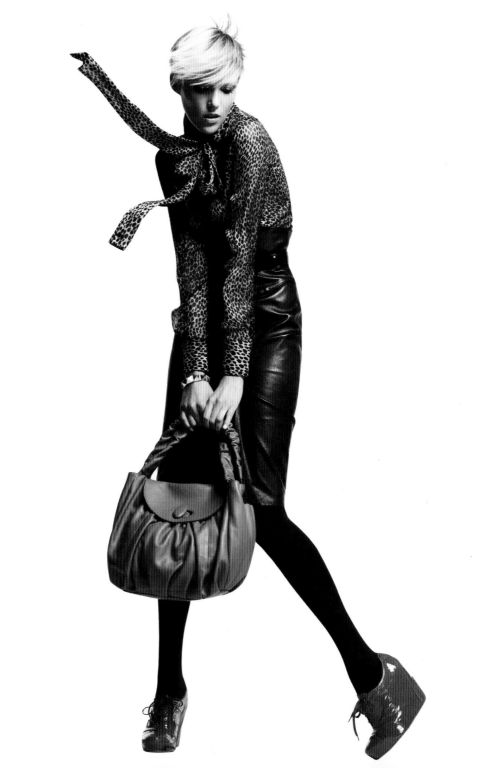

CHAPTER THREE

How to Wear It: Tops

Whatever your age and shape, there's a wonderful world of tops meant just for you. But picking one can be like selecting the right paint color—it's hard to choose from so many great options. So make smart choices and go for those that suit your personality and lifestyle

{ "You can be the chicest thing in the world in a T-shirt and jeans—it's up to you." —KARL LAGERFELD }

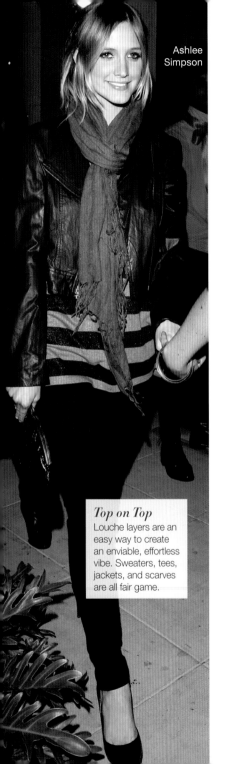

Ashlee
Simpson

Top on Top
Louche layers are an
easy way to create
an enviable, effortless
vibe. Sweaters, tees,
jackets, and scarves
are all fair game.

{ 20s }

Tops are the anchor to a great wardrobe. Start
with the basics and add more daring pieces

• **Layer them.** At any age, simple tops are terrific pieces to just grab
on the fly and pile on, whether you're actually in a rush or you're
going for a deliberate laid-back look. Start with T-shirts or tanks and
then add a cardigan or jacket—or both. Pair with jeans for
weekends or a slim skirt for the office.

• **Go bold with a sweater that's more than just a cotton staple**.
A smattering of shiny sequins or a shredded, weblike knit can
spice up daytime ensembles.

• **Prim and princess-y can be sexy when it's done right.** Let a slim
skirt, shorts, or a skinny pant play counterpoint to the sweetness
of a girlish frill or Peter Pan collar. To be truly daring, go sheer.

• **Balance a ladylike piece with something edgier.** A men's vest
tempers the loveliness of a blouse with a floppy bow. It looks
uptown with a skirt or downtown paired with jeans.

• **Drama is in the details of a flourish, a flounce, or a demonstrative
architectural detail.** Draw attention to your neckline with something
eye-catching, but keep your pants or skirt neutral and simple.

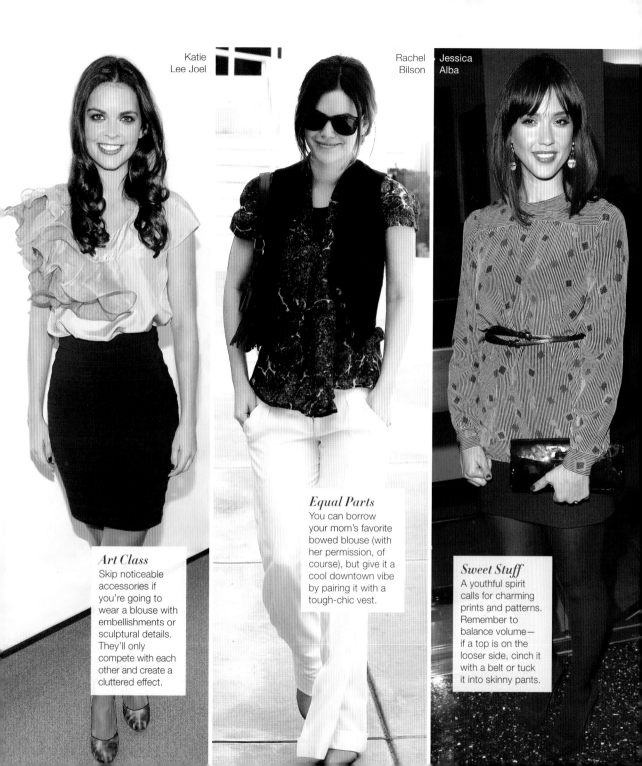

Katie
Lee Joel

Rachel
Bilson

Jessica
Alba

Art Class

Skip noticeable accessories if you're going to wear a blouse with embellishments or sculptural details. They'll only compete with each other and create a cluttered effect.

Equal Parts

You can borrow your mom's favorite bowed blouse (with her permission, of course), but give it a cool downtown vibe by pairing it with a tough-chic vest.

Sweet Stuff

A youthful spirit calls for charming prints and patterns. Remember to balance volume— if a top is on the looser side, cinch it with a belt or tuck it into skinny pants.

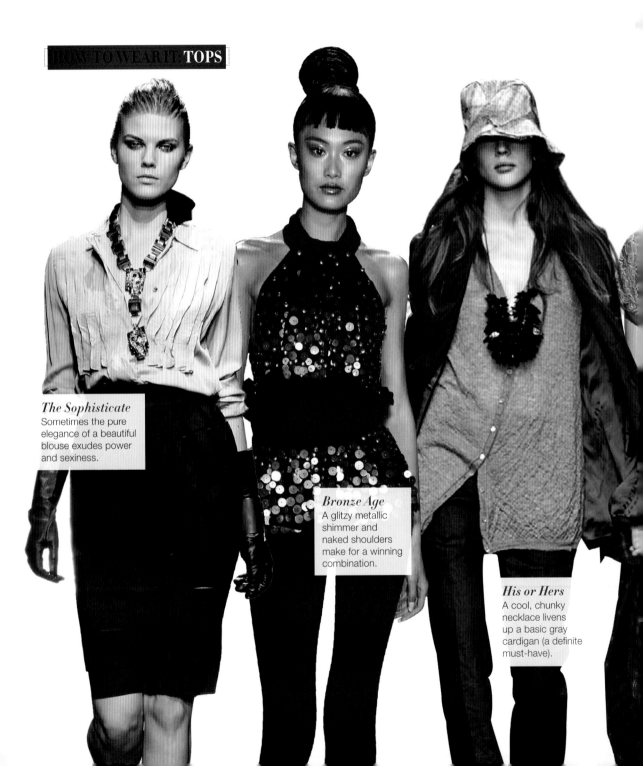

The Sophisticate
Sometimes the pure elegance of a beautiful blouse exudes power and sexiness.

Bronze Age
A glitzy metallic shimmer and naked shoulders make for a winning combination.

His or Hers
A cool, chunky necklace livens up a basic gray cardigan (a definite must-have).

Looks We Love

Play it any which way. Variety is the spice of life— and your wardrobe

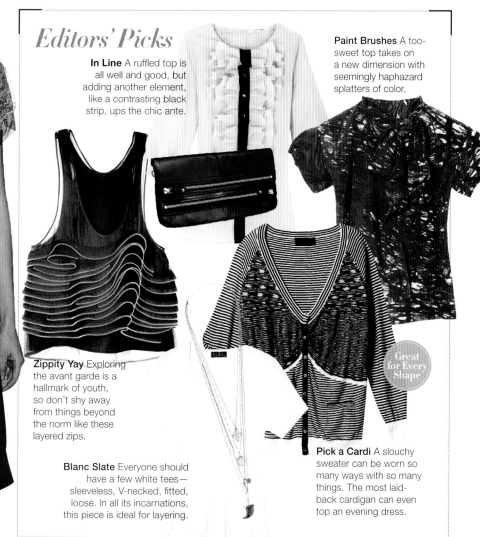

Editors' Picks

In Line A ruffled top is all well and good, but adding another element, like a contrasting black strip, ups the chic ante.

Paint Brushes A too-sweet top takes on a new dimension with seemingly haphazard splatters of color.

Zippity Yay Exploring the avant garde is a hallmark of youth, so don't shy away from things beyond the norm like these layered zips.

Blanc Slate Everyone should have a few white tees— sleeveless, V-necked, fitted, loose. In all its incarnations, this piece is ideal for layering.

Pick a Cardi A slouchy sweater can be worn so many ways with so many things. The most laid-back cardigan can even top an evening dress.

Great for Every Shape

Feel This
If you're not into poppy prints and patterns, texture is a great way to add interest.

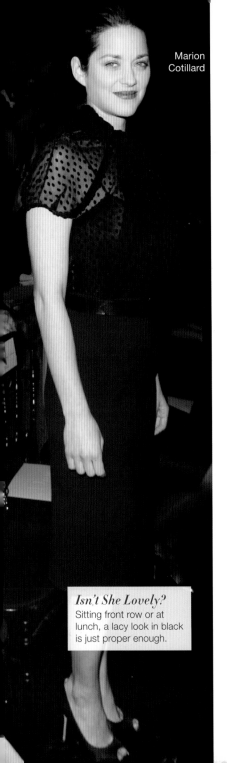

Marion
Cotillard

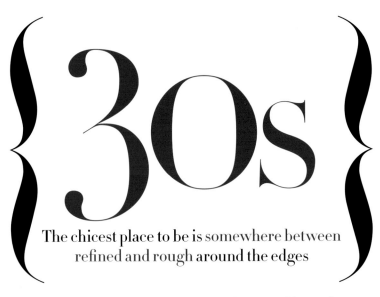

{ 30s }

The chicest place to be is somewhere between
refined and rough around the edges

Isn't She Lovely?
Sitting front row or at
lunch, a lacy look in black
is just proper enough.

• **A white button-down shirt is for the boardroom and beyond.**
Buy one now and keep it forever. Accessorize a minimal one
with bold necklaces, or go for a fitted, menswear style.

• **The plain white tee is the LBD of tops.** It's the sartorial blank
canvas. Stock up on short-sleeve versions and white-ribbed tanks
(or swipe them from your boyfriend's drawer). They layer with
other tops and sweaters beautifully but can also stand on their
own with jeans. V-necks look great on bustier girls and boyish
figures alike.

• **Mister Rogers was a style arbiter, slipping into his cardigan every
day.** Buttoned up and belted or left loose to hang, this sweater
is a must-have. Pick them in any color of cotton or cashmere.

• **Tops have a secret life—as dresses.** Opt for an extra-long or
extra-big look and it can double as a mini. But be aware of what
length looks right for you.

• **You're all grown up, and so you need a few pretty blouses
that skew toward ladylike.** They come in handy for last-minute
interviews or for holiday dos with the family.

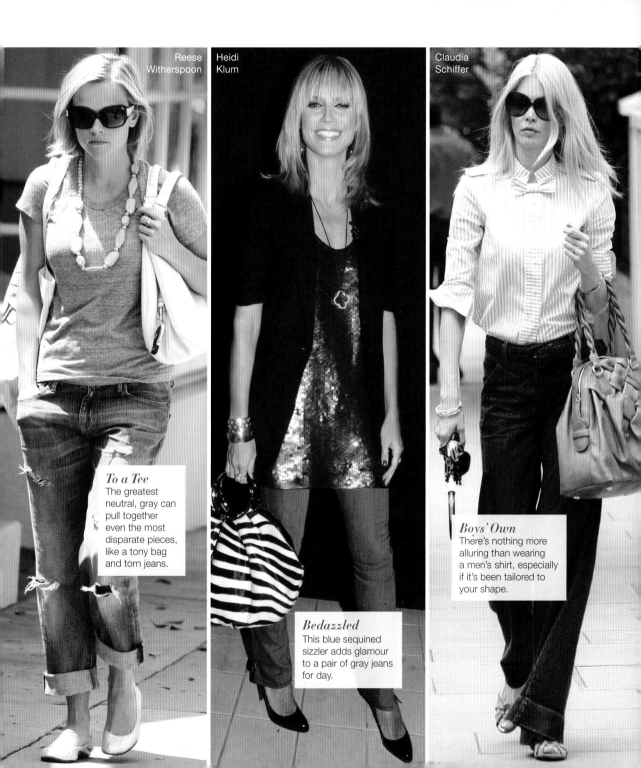

Reese Witherspoon

Heidi Klum

Claudia Schiffer

To a Tee
The greatest neutral, gray can pull together even the most disparate pieces, like a tony bag and torn jeans.

Bedazzled
This blue sequined sizzler adds glamour to a pair of gray jeans for day.

Boys' Own
There's nothing more alluring than wearing a men's shirt, especially if it's been tailored to your shape.

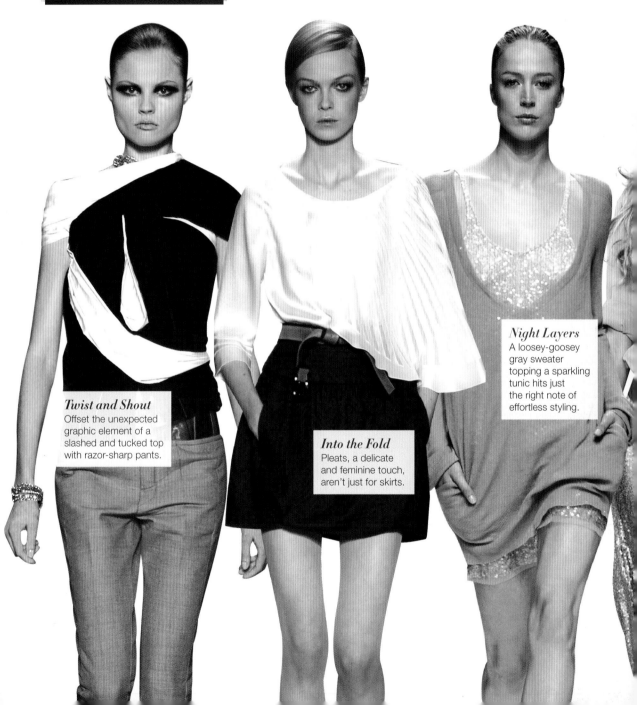

Twist and Shout
Offset the unexpected graphic element of a slashed and tucked top with razor-sharp pants.

Into the Fold
Pleats, a delicate and feminine touch, aren't just for skirts.

Night Layers
A loosey-goosey gray sweater topping a sparkling tunic hits just the right note of effortless styling.

Looks We Love

Pick tops and tees that will add snap, crackle, and pop to your wardrobe

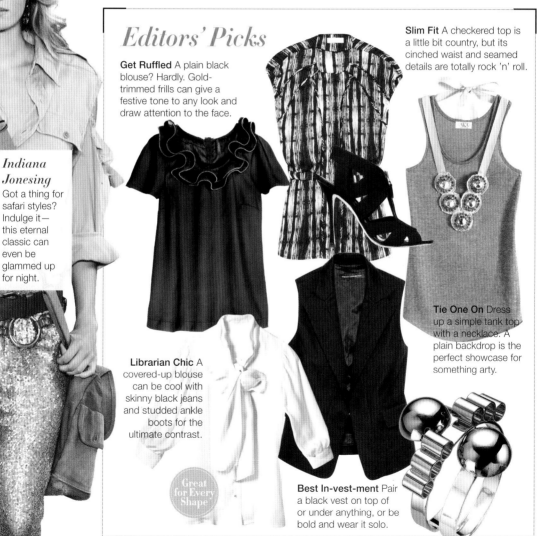

Editors' Picks

Get Ruffled A plain black blouse? Hardly. Gold-trimmed frills can give a festive tone to any look and draw attention to the face.

Indiana Jonesing Got a thing for safari styles? Indulge it—this eternal classic can even be glammed up for night.

Slim Fit A checkered top is a little bit country, but its cinched waist and seamed details are totally rock 'n' roll.

Tie One On Dress up a simple tank top with a necklace. A plain backdrop is the perfect showcase for something arty.

Librarian Chic A covered-up blouse can be cool with skinny black jeans and studded ankle boots for the ultimate contrast.

Great for Every Shape

Best In-vest-ment Pair a black vest on top of or under anything, or be bold and wear it solo.

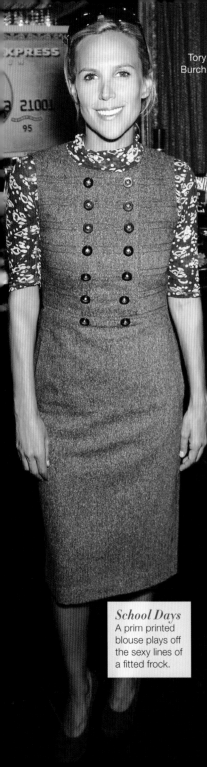

Tory
Burch

School Days
A prim printed
blouse plays off
the sexy lines of
a fitted frock.

{40s}

Your collection of tops, like your 401(k), should be diversified

• **Feathers and fringe, oh my!** You can pull off a dramatic collar of the fluffy stuff—even for day. Just keep it trim, tasteful, and discreet and tone down everything else.

• **Move beyond skimpy and flimsy blouses and tees.** Visible bra straps and other unmentionables are an absolute no-no. If you do go sheer, keep it covered with a delicate, lovely camisole.

• **Girlish is still good to go.** Frilled and ruffled skirts can read too young—and can also be unforgiving on hips of any age. Frilled and ruffled blouses, however, are simply stunning.

• **This is the age of the strong shoulder.** An exaggerated shoulder courtesy of structure—not pads—delivers a subtle air of assurance.

• **Understatement is hip, too.** Paring it back to a plain shirt or monochrome layers lets your hard-earned confidence shine through. You've learned that your clothes never wear you.

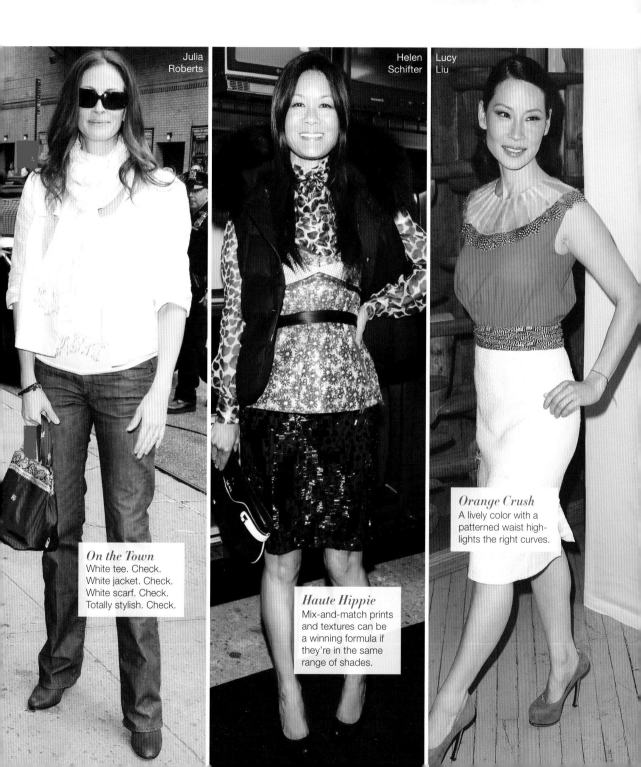

Julia
Roberts

Helen
Schifter

Lucy
Liu

Orange Crush
A lively color with a
patterned waist high-
lights the right curves.

On the Town
White tee. Check.
White jacket. Check.
White scarf. Check.
Totally stylish. Check.

Haute Hippie
Mix-and-match prints
and textures can be
a winning formula if
they're in the same
range of shades.

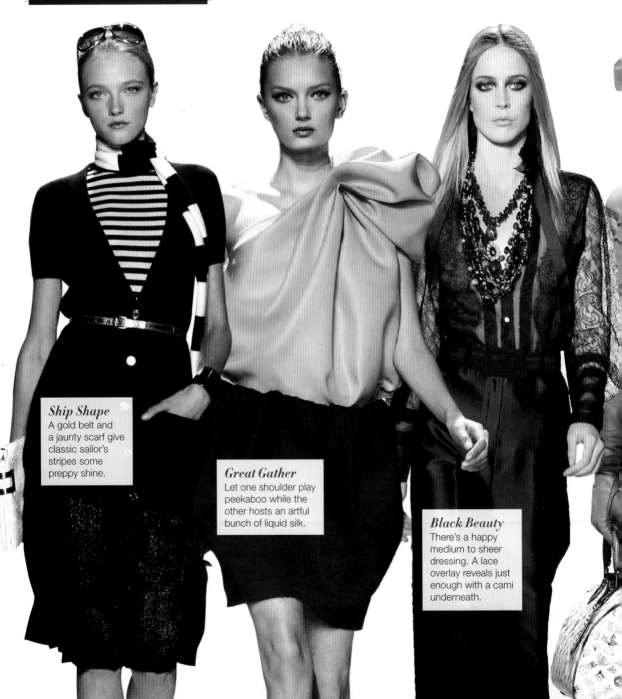

Ship Shape
A gold belt and a jaunty scarf give classic sailor's stripes some preppy shine.

Great Gather
Let one shoulder play peekaboo while the other hosts an artful bunch of liquid silk.

Black Beauty
There's a happy medium to sheer dressing. A lace overlay reveals just enough with a cami underneath.

Looks We Love

Let a great top be the crowning glory of your ensemble

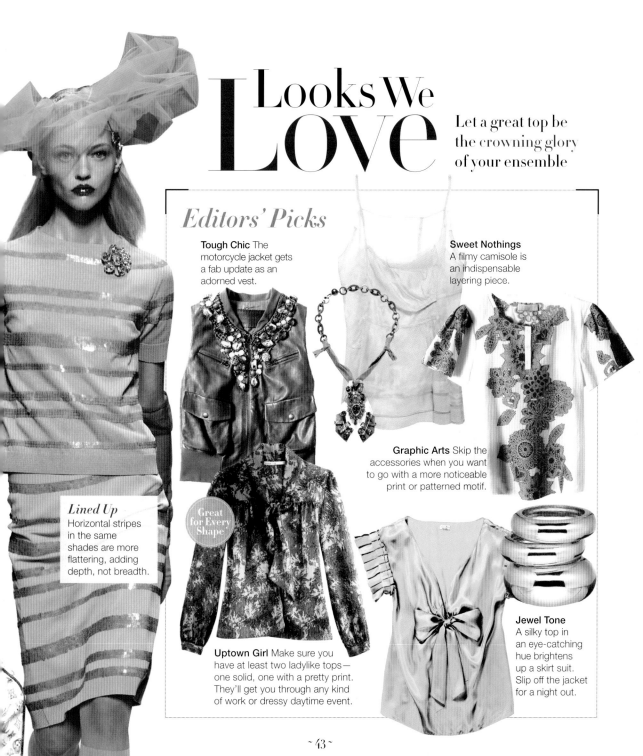

Editors' Picks

Tough Chic The motorcycle jacket gets a fab update as an adorned vest.

Sweet Nothings A filmy camisole is an indispensable layering piece.

Graphic Arts Skip the accessories when you want to go with a more noticeable print or patterned motif.

Great for Every Shape

Lined Up Horizontal stripes in the same shades are more flattering, adding depth, not breadth.

Uptown Girl Make sure you have at least two ladylike tops— one solid, one with a pretty print. They'll get you through any kind of work or dressy daytime event.

Jewel Tone A silky top in an eye-catching hue brightens up a skirt suit. Slip off the jacket for a night out.

{50s}

Brimming with confidence, you are always the epitome of put-together. That said, you know how to be adventurous, too

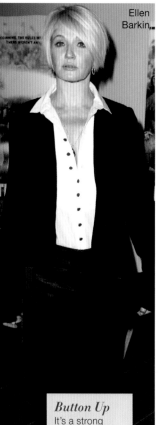

Ellen Barkin

• **Stock up on powerful patterns.** Graphics, polka dots, tie-dyes, florals, and abstracts all pack a punch. Animal prints spice up tops, and the natural color palette plays well with others.

• **"Know your colors" is a rule that bears repeating.** By now, you're aware of what you should avoid. The wrong shade can add ten years, while the right one will make your hair and eyes pop.

• **If you're proud of your biceps, triceps, and delts, by all means show them off.** But if you haven't been able to visit the gym in a while, a three-quarter-length sleeve hides a multitude of sins.

• **A men's shirt is a must.** There are plenty of options for a button-down shirt. Undoing the first three closures uncovers a tempting hint of skin.

Button Up
It's a strong woman who can carry off a spare white shirt for evening. You can do it.

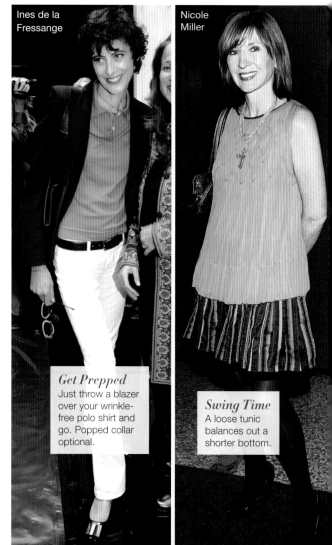

Ines de la Fressange

Nicole Miller

Get Prepped
Just throw a blazer over your wrinkle-free polo shirt and go. Popped collar optional.

Swing Time
A loose tunic balances out a shorter bottom.

Looks We Love

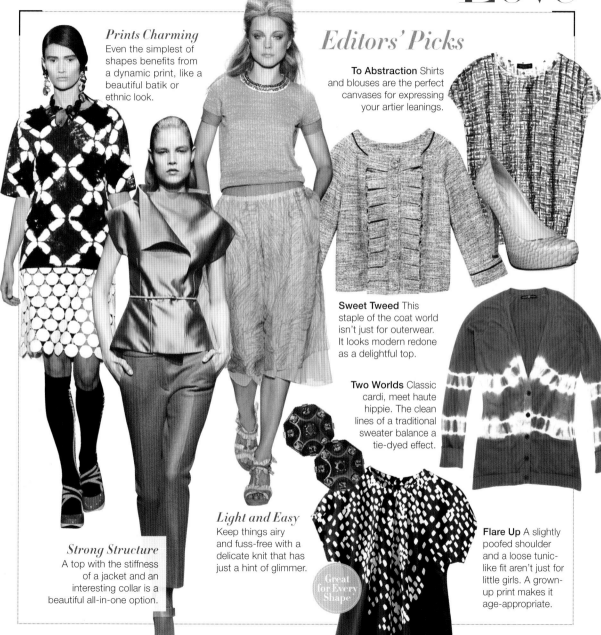

Editors' Picks

Prints Charming
Even the simplest of shapes benefits from a dynamic print, like a beautiful batik or ethnic look.

To Abstraction Shirts and blouses are the perfect canvases for expressing your artier leanings.

Sweet Tweed This staple of the coat world isn't just for outerwear. It looks modern redone as a delightful top.

Two Worlds Classic cardi, meet haute hippie. The clean lines of a traditional sweater balance a tie-dyed effect.

Strong Structure
A top with the stiffness of a jacket and an interesting collar is a beautiful all-in-one option.

Light and Easy
Keep things airy and fuss-free with a delicate knit that has just a hint of glimmer.

Great for Every Shape

Flare Up A slightly poofed shoulder and a loose tunic-like fit aren't just for little girls. A grown-up print makes it age-appropriate.

~ 45 ~

{60s}

You've got the know-how to reinvent a range of options for any occasion

• **There's an art to making a simple shirt**—or even a plain cotton undershirt—look like a million. But understatement mixed with a little moxie makes for something special.

• **Mix your motifs.** Pair shine with matte, silky with rough-hewn, flimsy with substantial.

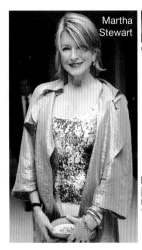

Martha Stewart

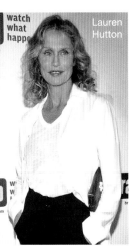

watch what happe

Lauren Hutton

Sequined Sass
A spangled tank or T-shirt is just the thing to brighten up any daytime event.

Tee Zone
There's nothing more fabulously confident than wearing a men's T-shirt for a night out.

{70+}

Grace and poise are the hallmarks of your blouses and sweaters

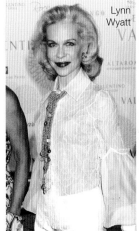

Lynn Wyatt

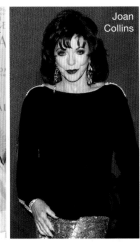

Joan Collins

Poetic License
Bold beads paired with the palest lace—for evening it's all about impact.

Back in Black
Smartly placed sequins or rhinestones give a petite frame more proportion.

• **Dramatic gestures can come in many forms:** a ruffled collar, a fluted sleeve, a whisper-thin layer of lace, a sizzling dash of color. Wear what best suits your mood.

• **Know when to keep things hushed.** The secret to style is understanding when enough is enough and when to lighten up on all those awesome details. Remember, a pristine ironed shirt can be the most successful look of all.

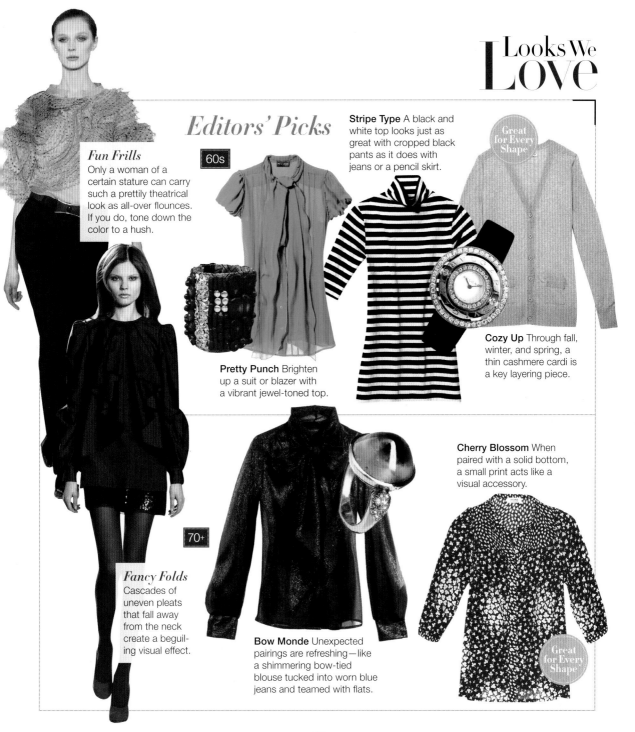

Editors' Picks

Fun Frills
Only a woman of a certain stature can carry such a prettily theatrical look as all-over flounces. If you do, tone down the color to a hush.

60s

Stripe Type A black and white top looks just as great with cropped black pants as it does with jeans or a pencil skirt.

Great for Every Shape

Pretty Punch Brighten up a suit or blazer with a vibrant jewel-toned top.

Cozy Up Through fall, winter, and spring, a thin cashmere cardi is a key layering piece.

70+

Fancy Folds
Cascades of uneven pleats that fall away from the neck create a beguiling visual effect.

Cherry Blossom When paired with a solid bottom, a small print acts like a visual accessory.

Bow Monde Unexpected pairings are refreshing—like a shimmering bow-tied blouse tucked into worn blue jeans and teamed with flats.

Great for Every Shape

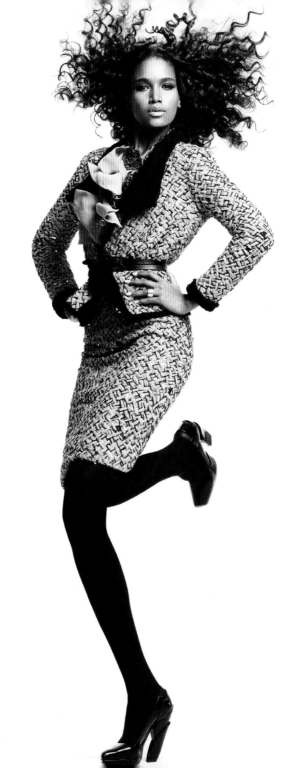

CHAPTER FOUR

How to Wear It: Skirts

Every great wardrobe should be anchored by an eclectic
set of skirts of the perfect shape and length. A few versatile pieces
can be styled any which way to suit many moods: saucy, serious,
dressed up, relaxed, girlish, or soigné

{ "After a certain age, you should
not wear too short or too girly.
I wear what feels comfortable
and what maintains an agile
silhouette." —DIANE VON FURSTENBERG }

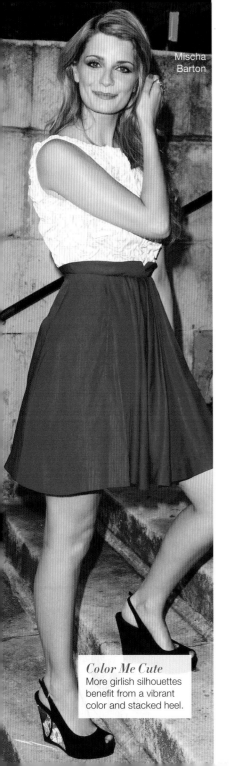

Mischa Barton

Color Me Cute
More girlish silhouettes benefit from a vibrant color and stacked heel.

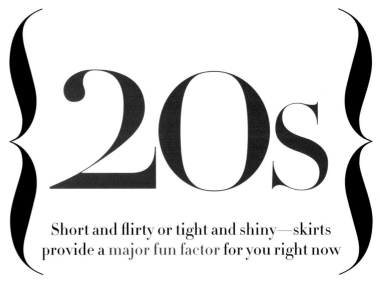

{20s}

Short and flirty or tight and shiny—skirts provide a major fun factor for you right now

• **Yes, short-short is OK.** If you have the legs to pull it off (and be brutally honest with yourself as to whether you do), a mini—or a micro-mini—is a must. You can even work the look in cooler months with tights and boots. Either way, to keep things balanced and chicly polite, don't go for too sexy a heel shape.

• **Opt for jazzier basics.** No matter what shape, size, or age, you can't go wrong with a pencil skirt. In addition to one in black (to pair with a white blouse, a slim knit, or a tank and heaps of chains), choose a bright color or metallic hue for a youthful edge.

• **Play with print and pattern.** A swath of broad cloth is the ideal canvas for brilliant, colorful motifs, whether you lean toward the arty and graphic or the hippie bohemian.

• **The 1950s were fab.** A pretty pouf, cinched with a belt or wide tab, is a great option for playing during the day or dressing up for the office. Tuck in a sweater, or keep it simple with a crisp tee. An exaggerated flare, though, should never creep above the knee or sink below midcalf.

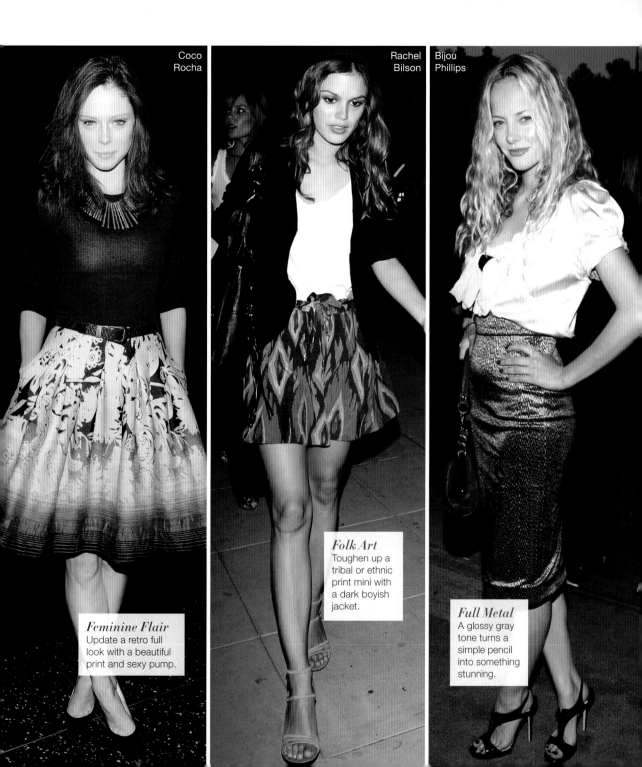

Coco
Rocha

Rachel
Bilson

Bijou
Phillips

Feminine Flair
Update a retro full
look with a beautiful
print and sexy pump.

Folk Art
Toughen up a
tribal or ethnic
print mini with
a dark boyish
jacket.

Full Metal
A glossy gray
tone turns a
simple pencil
into something
stunning.

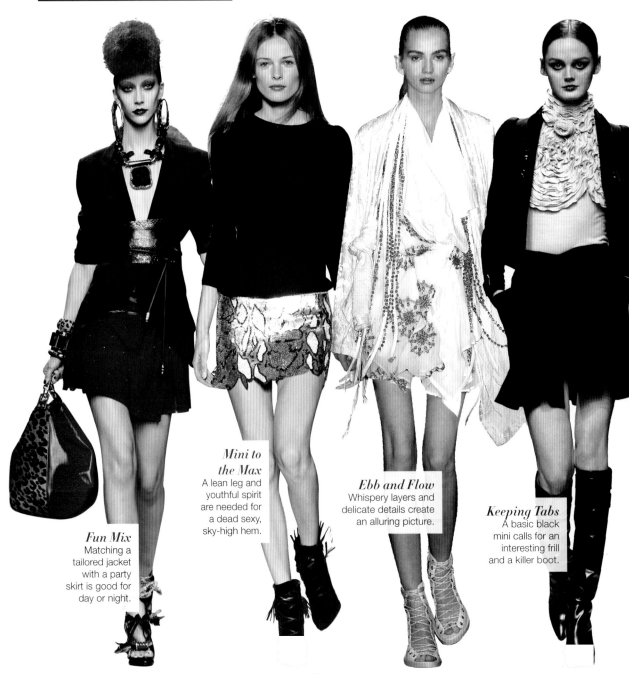

Fun Mix
Matching a
tailored jacket
with a party
skirt is good for
day or night.

**Mini to
the Max**
A lean leg and
youthful spirit
are needed for
a dead sexy,
sky-high hem.

Ebb and Flow
Whispery layers and
delicate details create
an alluring picture.

Keeping Tabs
A basic black
mini calls for an
interesting frill
and a killer boot.

Looks We Love

A fun, fantastic piece can be the chic focal point of any ensemble

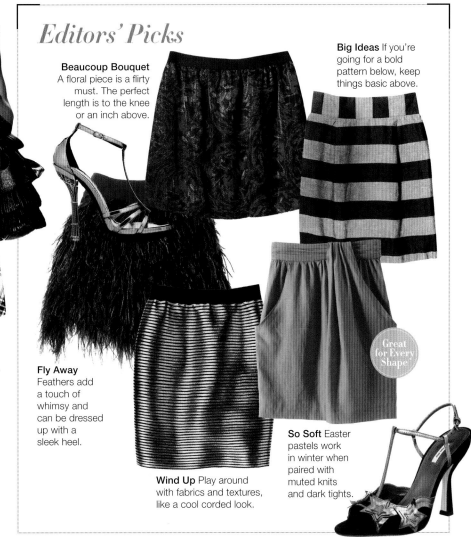

Editors' Picks

Beaucoup Bouquet
A floral piece is a flirty must. The perfect length is to the knee or an inch above.

Big Ideas If you're going for a bold pattern below, keep things basic above.

Fly Away
Feathers add a touch of whimsy and can be dressed up with a sleek heel.

Wind Up Play around with fabrics and textures, like a cool corded look.

Great for Every Shape

So Soft Easter pastels work in winter when paired with muted knits and dark tights.

Check This
Plaid isn't just for the office— an oversized version can be fun and laidback.

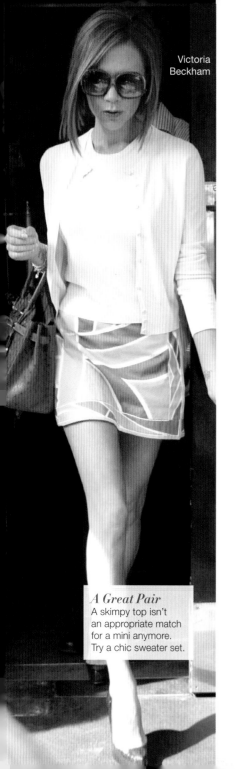

Victoria
Beckham

A Great Pair
A skimpy top isn't
an appropriate match
for a mini anymore.
Try a chic sweater set.

{ 30s }

A day-to-night staple, the right skirt is
the ultimate accessory for style mavens

• **Any length will do (almost!).** You're on the tail end of being able
to get away with some of the über-short lengths out there (again,
be honest about what you can carry off). But a mid-to-lower-thigh
hem is perfect. And now you can wear a sleek, long ankle-grazer—
without looking like you're playing dress-up.

• **Slouched to perfection.** A slightly rumpled effect has neat street
appeal and can even make it to the office if your top, shoes, and
coif are impeccable.

• **Invest in precious metals.** Stocking up on 24-karat gold and
jeweled baubles might not be a fiscal reality yet, but you can still
live rich in gold, silver, and bronzed metallic skirts.

• **Get all aflutter.** Nothing says feminine like a well-placed flounce,
ruffle, or tier. But to avoid looking 30 going on 13, make sure there
isn't too much flou.

• **Structural effects can be as striking as a major accessory.** A
series of pleats or a flap can look sensational as long as they fall
below the hip.

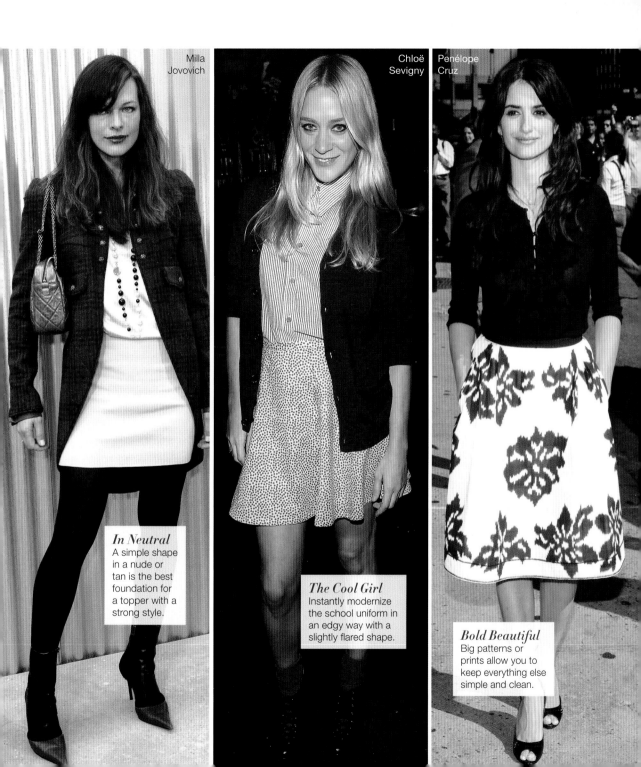

Milla
Jovovich

Chloë
Sevigny

Penélope
Cruz

In Neutral
A simple shape
in a nude or
tan is the best
foundation for
a topper with a
strong style.

The Cool Girl
Instantly modernize
the school uniform in
an edgy way with a
slightly flared shape.

Bold Beautiful
Big patterns or
prints allow you to
keep everything else
simple and clean.

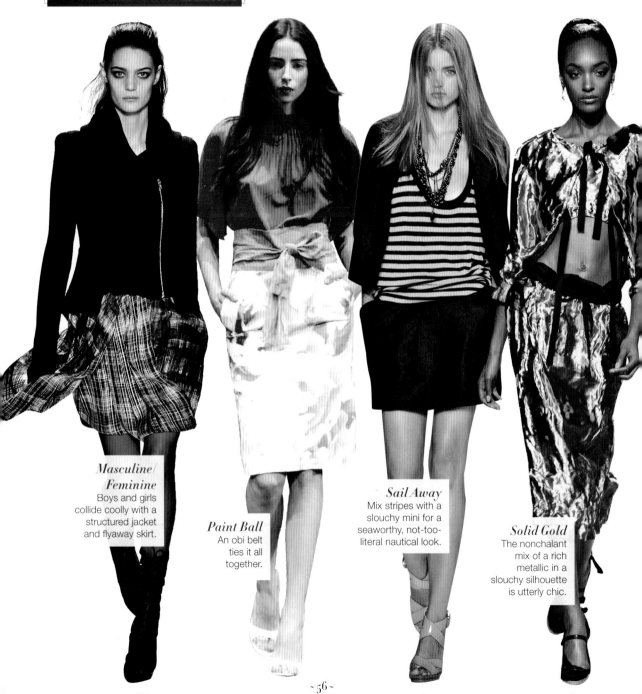

*Masculine/
Feminine*
Boys and girls
collide coolly with a
structured jacket
and flyaway skirt.

Paint Ball
An obi belt
ties it all
together.

Sail Away
Mix stripes with a
slouchy mini for a
seaworthy, not-too-
literal nautical look.

Solid Gold
The nonchalant
mix of a rich
metallic in a
slouchy silhouette
is utterly chic.

Looks We Love

Add depth to your closet with dressed-up, colorful, textured pieces

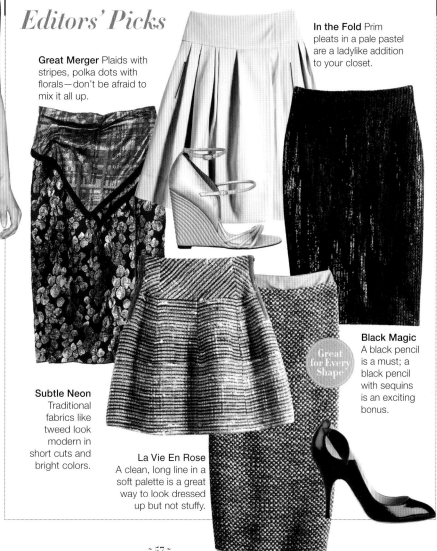

Go Long
A floor-length style in a dark hue will instantly elongate and slim your shape.

Editors' Picks

Great Merger Plaids with stripes, polka dots with florals—don't be afraid to mix it all up.

In the Fold Prim pleats in a pale pastel are a ladylike addition to your closet.

Subtle Neon Traditional fabrics like tweed look modern in short cuts and bright colors.

La Vie En Rose A clean, long line in a soft palette is a great way to look dressed up but not stuffy.

Great for Every Shape

Black Magic A black pencil is a must; a black pencil with sequins is an exciting bonus.

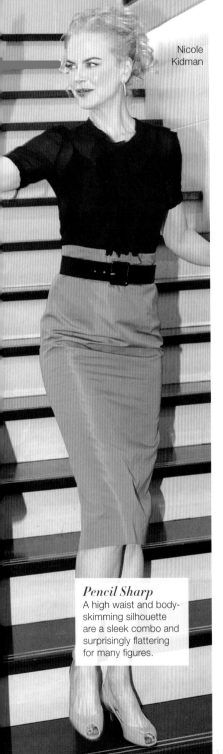

Nicole Kidman

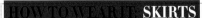

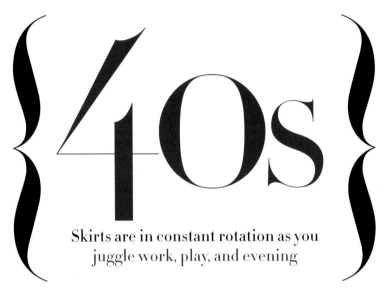

{4Os}

Skirts are in constant rotation as you juggle work, play, and evening

- **How low can you go?** If you're petite, longer lengths can swallow you up. Try to keep hems at the knee or just an inch above. If you're tall, minis and cropped looks can make your legs look disproportionately longer than your torso, so a natural or dropped waist is advisable.

- **Think about separates for evening.** You may have collected quite a lineup of evening dresses and party frocks, but a skirt is a sophisticated, fashion-forward option for soirees.

- **From office to party.** The same skirt can be transformed with smart accessory choices. A long chain and a higher heel (perhaps strappy) will transform your outfit. Likewise, change your leather belt for a gold or patent cincher. And nothing says nighttime like bare legs.

- **Curves or straight ahead?** Boxy shapes will do nothing for slim, boyish figures, but defined waists, pleats, and layers will. And if you've got curves, dark solids, tight patterns, and tailored lines will camouflage just about anything.

- **One skirt to rule them all.** The pencil skirt flatters everyone. Choose fit, pattern, and material based on what works for you.

Pencil Sharp
A high waist and body-skimming silhouette are a sleek combo and surprisingly flattering for many figures.

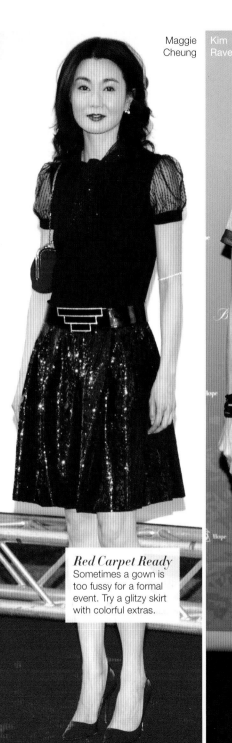

Maggie Cheung

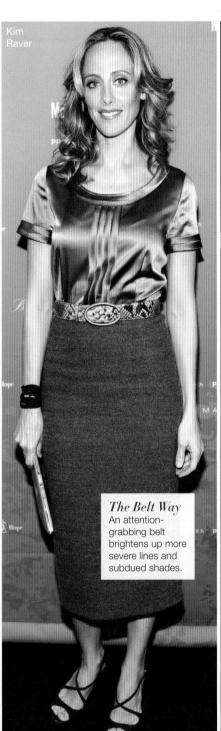

Kim Raver

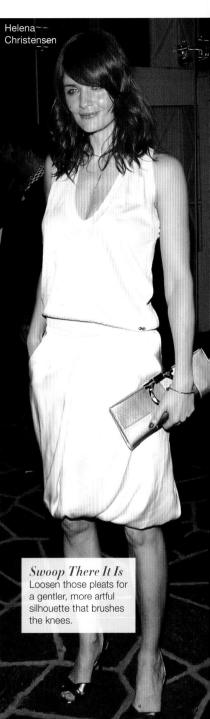

Helena Christensen

Red Carpet Ready
Sometimes a gown is too fussy for a formal event. Try a glitzy skirt with colorful extras.

The Belt Way
An attention-grabbing belt brightens up more severe lines and subdued shades.

Swoop There It Is
Loosen those pleats for a gentler, more artful silhouette that brushes the knees.

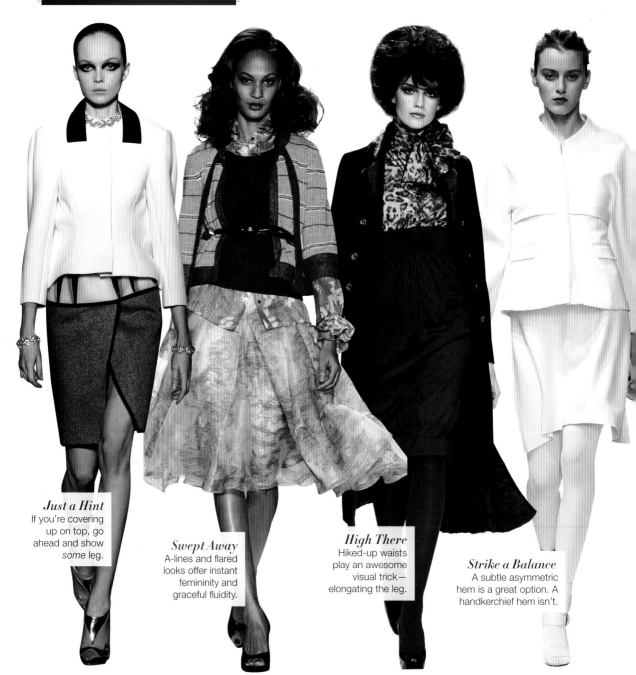

Just a Hint
If you're covering up on top, go ahead and show *some* leg.

Swept Away
A-lines and flared looks offer instant femininity and graceful fluidity.

High There
Hiked-up waists play an awesome visual trick— elongating the leg.

Strike a Balance
A subtle asymmetric hem is a great option. A handkerchief hem isn't.

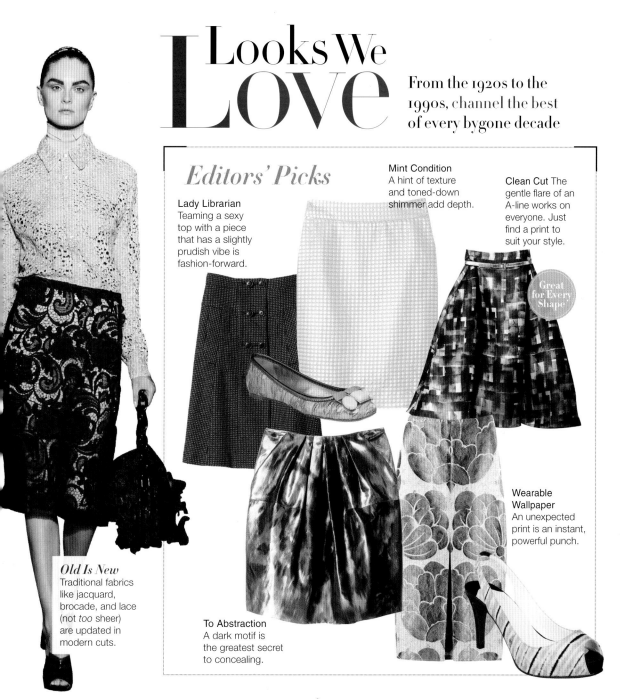

Looks We Love

From the 1920s to the 1990s, channel the best of every bygone decade

Editors' Picks

Lady Librarian
Teaming a sexy top with a piece that has a slightly prudish vibe is fashion-forward.

Mint Condition
A hint of texture and toned-down shimmer add depth.

Clean Cut The gentle flare of an A-line works on everyone. Just find a print to suit your style.

Great for Every Shape

Old Is New
Traditional fabrics like jacquard, brocade, and lace (not *too* sheer) are updated in modern cuts.

To Abstraction
A dark motif is the greatest secret to concealing.

Wearable Wallpaper
An unexpected print is an instant, powerful punch.

{50s}

Elegant, classic, and sophisticated are definitely far from boring—just the opposite, in fact

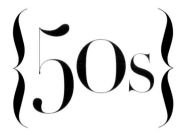

Joan Allen

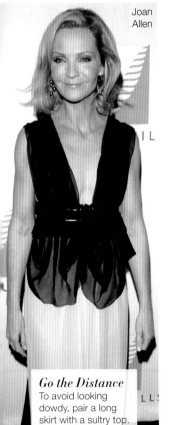

Go the Distance
To avoid looking dowdy, pair a long skirt with a sultry top.

• **Indulge in ladylike luxe.** Total uptown tony-ness doesn't always work when you're on the younger side of 50, but now you own that rich, well-shod look. Throw on pearls to complement an array of skirts in silk, lace, brocade, jacquard, and other sumptuous materials.

• **You can have it all.** In the battle between sex appeal and restraint, you win. The key is in mastering the delicate balance of working both at the same time.

• **For once, matchmaking works.** A great skirt suit is an easy way to dress that doesn't compromise an inch of style.

• **Follow the curve.** A well-fitting skirt is the simplest way to show off what God gave you. But remember that skintight is kind to no one.

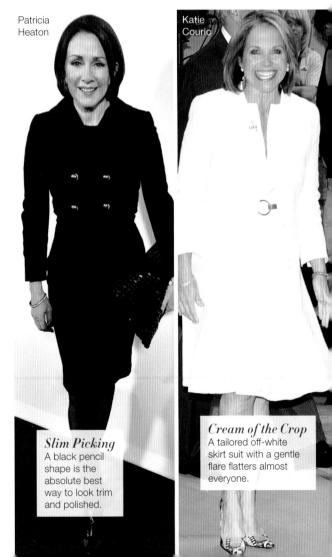

Patricia Heaton

Katie Couric

Slim Picking
A black pencil shape is the absolute best way to look trim and polished.

Cream of the Crop
A tailored off-white skirt suit with a gentle flare flatters almost everyone.

Looks We Love

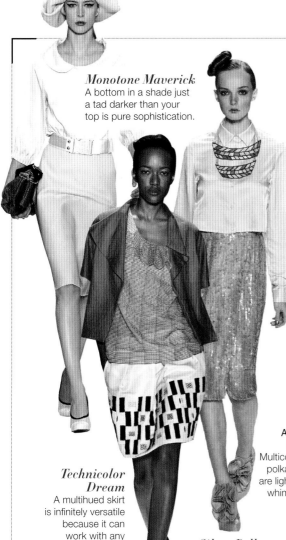

Monotone Maverick
A bottom in a shade just a tad darker than your top is pure sophistication.

Technicolor Dream
A multihued skirt is infinitely versatile because it can work with any number of tops.

Silver Belle
If you're not keen on top-to-toe sequins, how about a skirt to keep things glam?

Editors' Picks

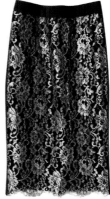

A Fine Line Adding a tuxedo stripe to a lace pattern print has a slimming effect.

Jungle Beat Every woman should own something in an animal print. It gives a skirt wow factor.

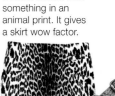

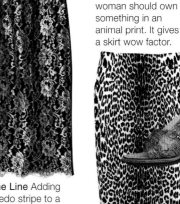

A Little Levity Multicolored polka dots are light and whimsical.

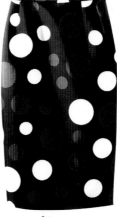

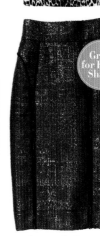

Great for Every Shape

It Seams So Piping illustrates great workmanship *and* creates curves.

{60s}

Now you can flirt with fuller shapes and clean lines alike

• **Stay strong with graphic patterns.** They make striking statements, and in the right silhouette will accentuate the positive.

• **When in doubt, cinch it.** A belted look or one with a tab waist creates instant shape and contours on slim figures.

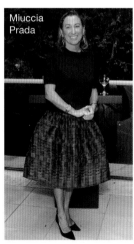

Miuccia Prada

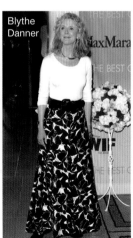

Blythe Danner

Red, Right, and Blue
Fresh color and pattern breathe new life into a playful dirndl skirt.

Long, Good Night
A voluminous skirt can be just as dramatic as a sweeping gown.

{70+}

You've collected an array of the basics—now break out the bold

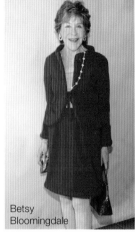

Betsy Bloomingdale

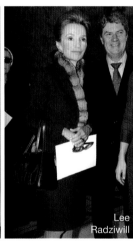

Lee Radziwill

Scarlet Fever
When opting for a punchy hue like cherry red, keep the shape sweet and simple.

Instant Chic
The ultimate in sophisticated day looks is an all-gray skirt suit with subtle detailing.

• **Don't skimp on color.** Cultivating a mixed palette is a great way to keep your closet adaptable to fashion's many moods. And you know what they say about variety being the spice of life.

• **Slouchy doesn't cut it anymore.** When it comes to dressing, make sure you dot your i's and cross your t's. Architectural details and razor-sharp tailoring (even on your most fluid of pieces) are the way to go.

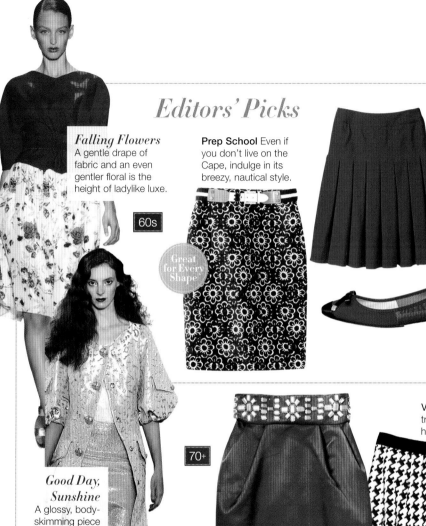

Editors' Picks

Falling Flowers
A gentle drape of fabric and an even gentler floral is the height of ladylike luxe.

60s

Prep School Even if you don't live on the Cape, indulge in its breezy, nautical style.

Great for Every Shape

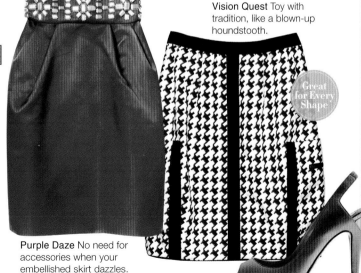

Prep to It Tons of tight pleats will put a kicky swing in your step.

Weave Got It Gray tweed is great as a neutral foil to poppy tops and vibrant accessories.

Good Day, Sunshine
A glossy, body-skimming piece is great for both layering and leaving alone.

70+

Vision Quest Toy with tradition, like a blown-up houndstooth.

Great for Every Shape

Purple Daze No need for accessories when your embellished skirt dazzles.

20s

30s

Skirt Suits

Once the uniform for only Ladies Who Lunch, these are now a staple for every well-dressed modern woman

On the Edge
Splicing traditional patterns makes for a fresh, modern look.

Max Mileage
Suits aren't meant just for the board-room. They can also be used as vibrant separates.

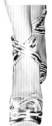

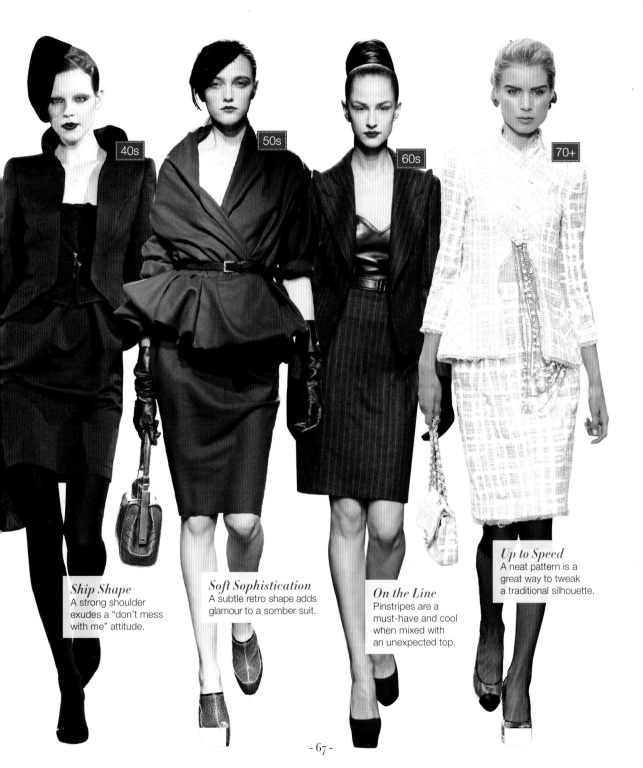

40s

50s

60s

70+

Ship Shape
A strong shoulder exudes a "don't mess with me" attitude.

Soft Sophistication
A subtle retro shape adds glamour to a somber suit.

On the Line
Pinstripes are a must-have and cool when mixed with an unexpected top.

Up to Speed
A neat pattern is a great way to tweak a traditional silhouette.

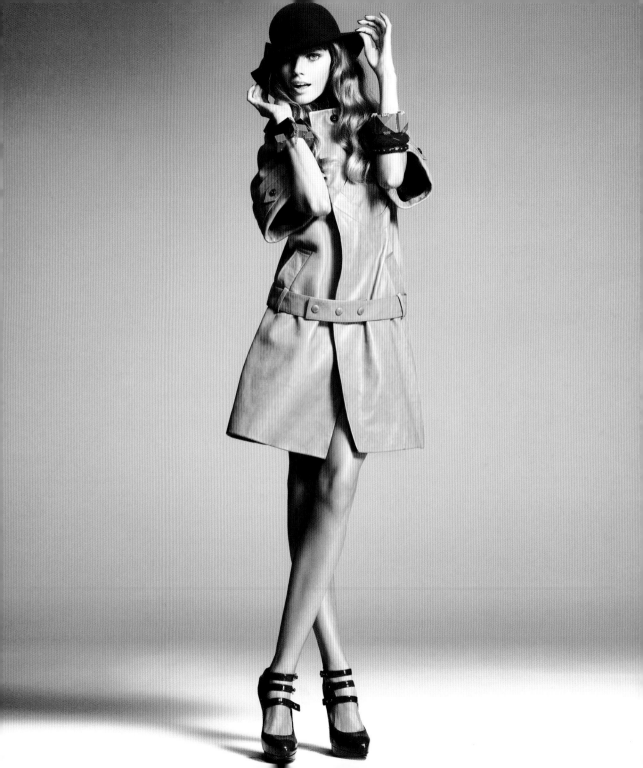

CHAPTER FIVE

How to Wear It: Jackets &Coats

Don't overlook these cover-ups as an exciting and easy way to update your closet. Remember, they're often the first thing people see. Plus, a good choice has serious staying power. Indulge yourself: There's everything from cheerful spring toppers to cool winter fare, big buys to bargains

{ "You know when something has longevity. When the proportions are right, the quality's perfect, and the creativity is strong." —DIEGO DELLA VALLE }

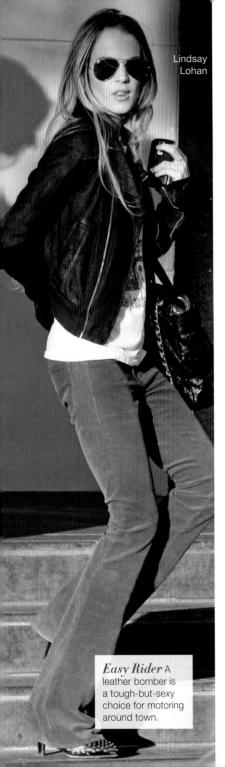

Lindsay Lohan

{20s}

Now is the time to channel your inner rock
star, coquette, or tomboy, depending on the day

• **Have fun.** If your 20s are a feast of fashion, then jackets and coats are your dessert. You need a few looks to get you through the seasons, and they're a sweet way to satisfy your need for variety: girly, tough, tailored, louche.

• **Join the boys' club.** A solid blazer (like the kind your dad wore in the 1980s) is a great investment. Throw it over a mini dress or a skinny pair of jeans.

• **Join the girls' club, too.** For dressier occasions, like a night at the theater or a holiday soiree, it helps to have one fantastically pretty, pulled-together long coat in wool or cashmere. A-lines or slightly fitted silhouettes stand the test of time (and are great for all figures).

• **Turn tradition on its head.** Everyone loves a trench, and you should, too. But if you desire something a little edgier, find one in a bright or unexpected color, studded with grommets, or embroidered. The same left-of-center approach is good for femme wool coats and classic blazers.

• **Let me hear you roar with a great animal print or bold graphic.** A fabulous jacket can be your statement piece. In that case, keep everything else simple so it doesn't steal the limelight.

Easy Rider A leather bomber is a tough-but-sexy choice for motoring around town.

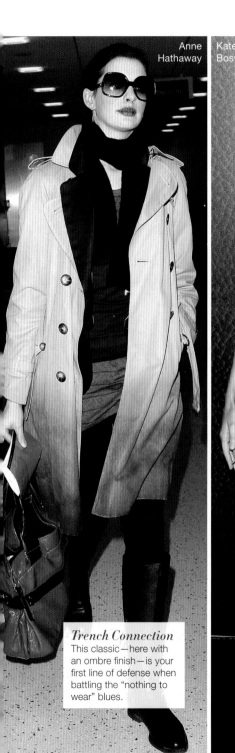

Anne Hathaway

Trench Connection
This classic—here with an ombre finish—is your first line of defense when battling the "nothing to wear" blues.

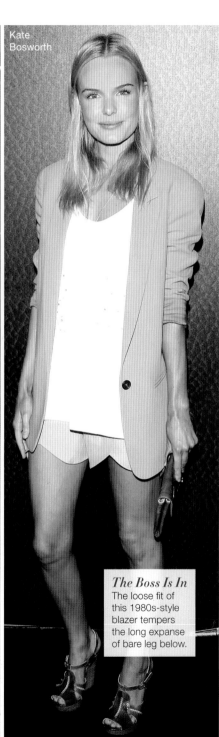

Kate Bosworth

The Boss Is In
The loose fit of this 1980s-style blazer tempers the long expanse of bare leg below.

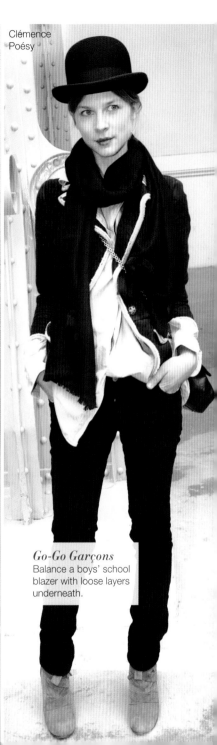

Clémence Poésy

Go-Go Garçons
Balance a boys' school blazer with loose layers underneath.

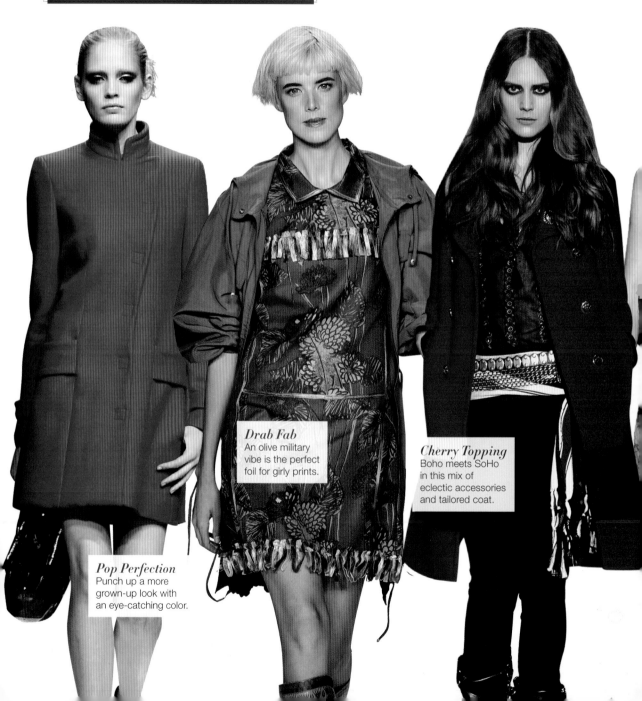

Drab Fab
An olive military
vibe is the perfect
foil for girly prints.

Cherry Topping
Boho meets SoHo
in this mix of
eclectic accessories
and tailored coat.

Pop Perfection
Punch up a more
grown-up look with
an eye-catching color.

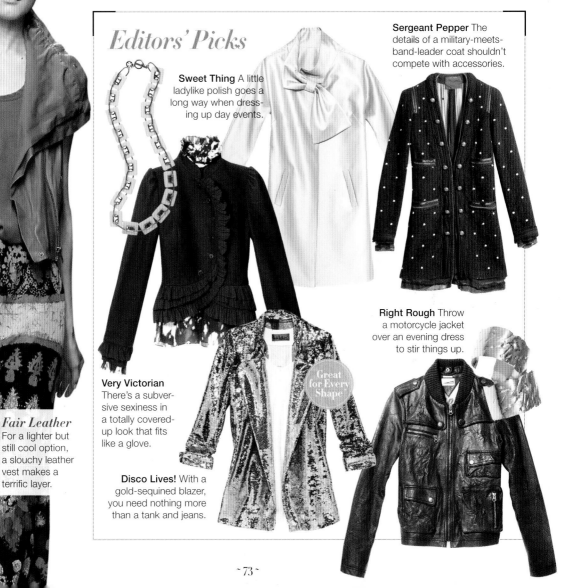

Looks We Love

Your outerwear should be a lively mix of flash, dash, and class, of course

Editors' Picks

Sweet Thing A little ladylike polish goes a long way when dressing up day events.

Sergeant Pepper The details of a military-meets-band-leader coat shouldn't compete with accessories.

Right Rough Throw a motorcycle jacket over an evening dress to stir things up.

Great for Every Shape

Very Victorian There's a subversive sexiness in a totally covered-up look that fits like a glove.

Disco Lives! With a gold-sequined blazer, you need nothing more than a tank and jeans.

Fair Leather For a lighter but still cool option, a slouchy leather vest makes a terrific layer.

{ 30s }

Increasingly, you're relying on looks that transform and accent your diverse wardrobe

• **Just ever-so-slightly over-the-top sounds and looks good right now.** The crazier, trendier styles should make way for more classic silhouettes that nevertheless still have plenty of interesting details.

• **A coat for all ages.** Toppers don't always come cheap, but a perfectly tailored look in a neutral tone and a good fabric will be as fabulous and wearable in a few years as it is at the moment.

• **Follow the same rules you would when trying on tops.** If you know a certain shape doesn't suit you, don't waste your time on a frustrating trip to the fitting room. Go straight to the cuts that flatter your figure. You know what they are by now.

• **From night to day.** There are some evening jackets, like a muted satin or silk number, that you can try on for day. You won't look at all wrong—just inventive.

• **It's like architecture.** Designers perform feats of wonder with interesting collars and layered effects that turn the tailored into the terrific.

• **Just belt it.** Even though it may sound antithetical to a coat's raison d'être, it's a clever styling trick to leave yours undone or slightly open but belted.

French Dressing
Sharp shoulders that segue into a cinched waist and belled skirt define Parisian chic.

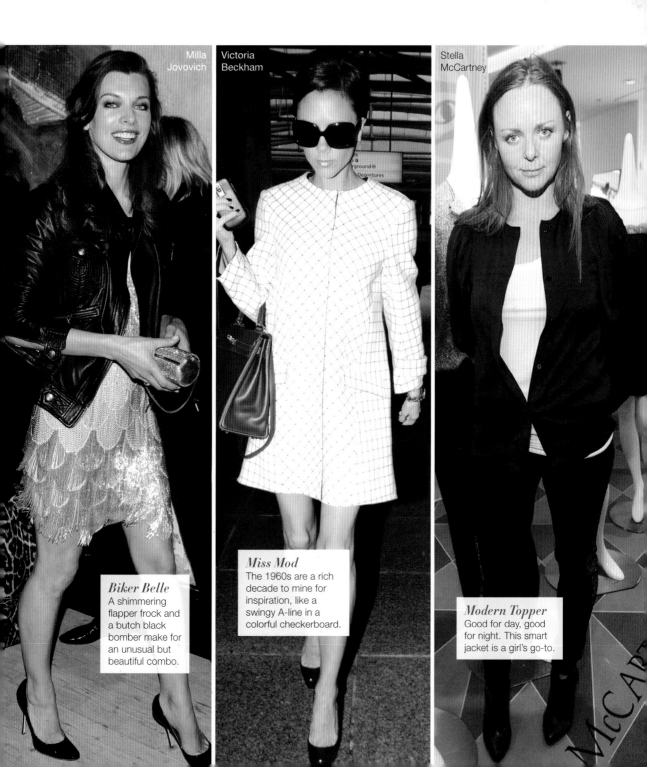

Milla Jovovich

Victoria Beckham

Stella McCartney

Biker Belle
A shimmering flapper frock and a butch black bomber make for an unusual but beautiful combo.

Miss Mod
The 1960s are a rich decade to mine for inspiration, like a swingy A-line in a colorful checkerboard.

Modern Topper
Good for day, good for night. This smart jacket is a girl's go-to.

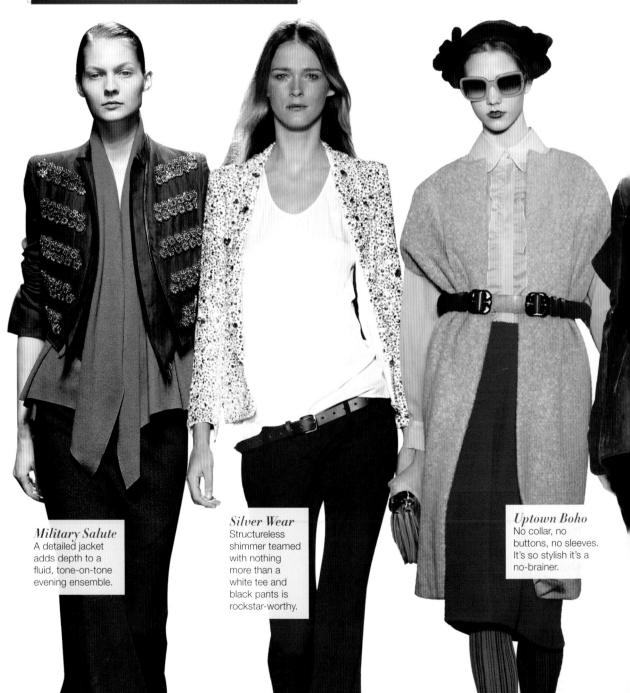

Military Salute
A detailed jacket adds depth to a fluid, tone-on-tone evening ensemble.

Silver Wear
Structureless shimmer teamed with nothing more than a white tee and black pants is rockstar-worthy.

Uptown Boho
No collar, no buttons, no sleeves. It's so stylish it's a no-brainer.

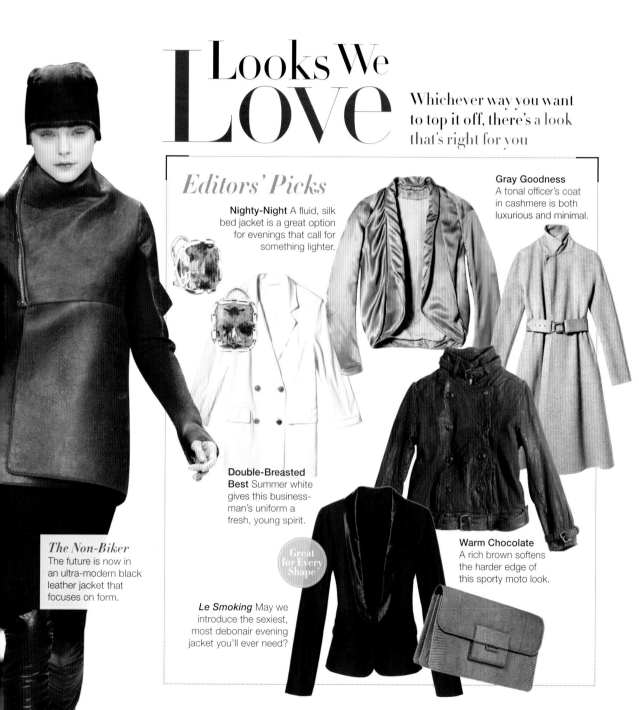

Looks We Love

Whichever way you want to top it off, there's a look that's right for you

Editors' Picks

Nighty-Night A fluid, silk bed jacket is a great option for evenings that call for something lighter.

Gray Goodness A tonal officer's coat in cashmere is both luxurious and minimal.

Double-Breasted Best Summer white gives this business-man's uniform a fresh, young spirit.

Warm Chocolate A rich brown softens the harder edge of this sporty moto look.

The Non-Biker The future is now in an ultra-modern black leather jacket that focuses on form.

Great for Every Shape

Le Smoking May we introduce the sexiest, most debonair evening jacket you'll ever need?

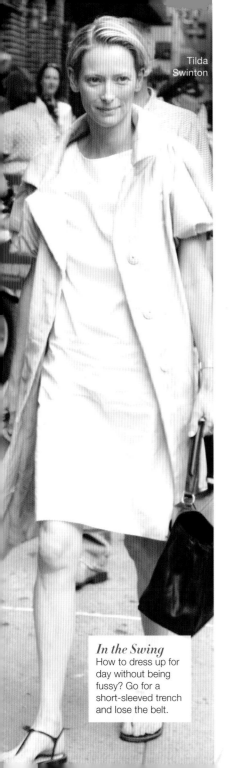

Tilda Swinton

In the Swing
How to dress up for day without being fussy? Go for a short-sleeved trench and lose the belt.

{ 40s }

The short and long (and in between) of it is that you can now pull off just about anything

• **The right topper can cover a multitude of sins.** A long belted look or jaunty swing version can hide the fact that you're totally dressed down underneath. This is a great way to still look put-together when you're just zipping out to buy groceries or hitting the movies.

• **Let your blazers come undone.** There's an appealing ease and languor to a structured look that's more relaxed than razor-sharp. It's meant for dressier occasions, though, not for the office. Pair with a body-conscious dress.

• **Luxe leathers are the way to go.** Store your studded motorcyclers for your daughter's rebellious years and go in for sleeker versions, perhaps in something other than black.

• **Mini, maxi, midi.** You came, you saw, you conquered all lengths. And when you open up your hall closet in the morning, you should be able to play eeny-meeny-miny-moe with all the great looks you've now amassed.

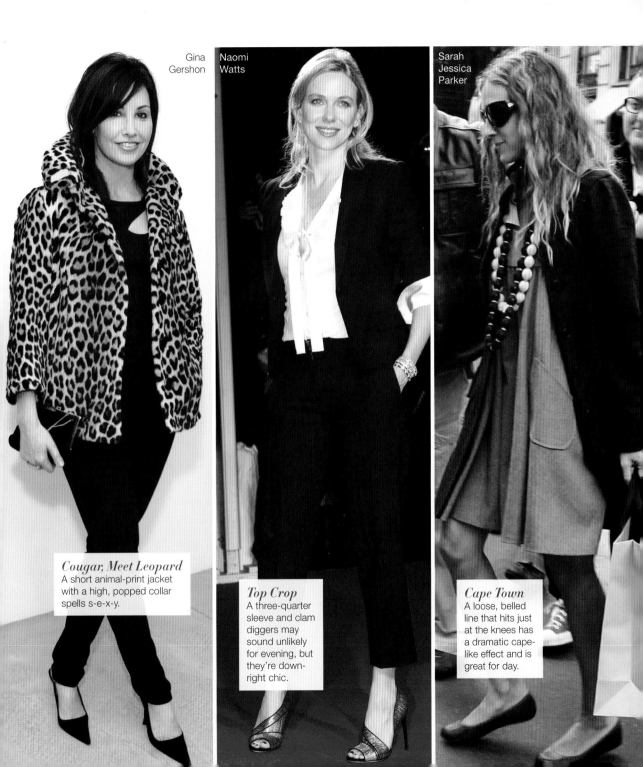

Gina
Gershon

Naomi
Watts

Sarah
Jessica
Parker

Cougar, Meet Leopard
A short animal-print jacket with a high, popped collar spells s-e-x-y.

Top Crop
A three-quarter sleeve and clam diggers may sound unlikely for evening, but they're down-right chic.

Cape Town
A loose, belled line that hits just at the knees has a dramatic cape-like effect and is great for day.

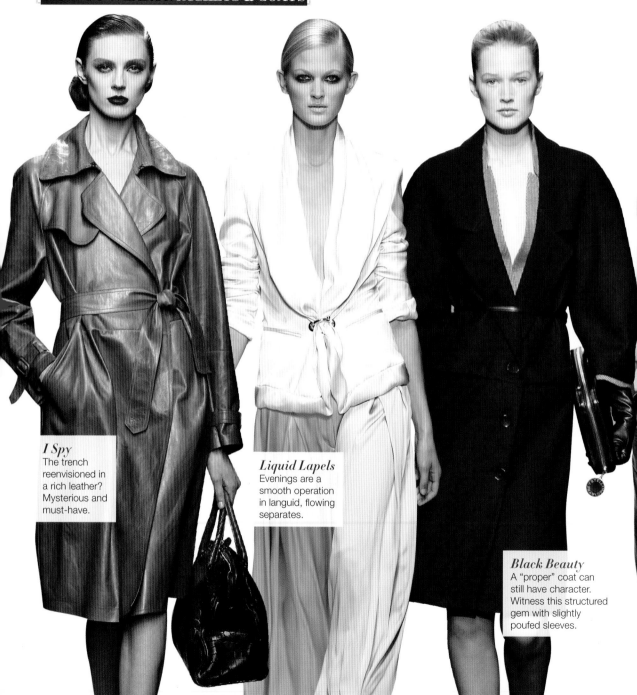

I Spy
The trench reenvisioned in a rich leather? Mysterious and must-have.

Liquid Lapels
Evenings are a smooth operation in languid, flowing separates.

Black Beauty
A "proper" coat can still have character. Witness this structured gem with slightly poufed sleeves.

Looks We Love

Whether tailored, belted, or loose, seek out classic pieces with unexpected touches

Editors' Picks

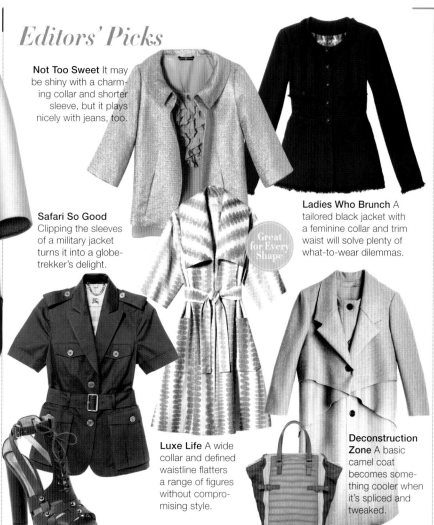

Not Too Sweet It may be shiny with a charming collar and shorter sleeve, but it plays nicely with jeans, too.

Safari So Good Clipping the sleeves of a military jacket turns it into a globe-trekker's delight.

Ladies Who Brunch A tailored black jacket with a feminine collar and trim waist will solve plenty of what-to-wear dilemmas.

Great for Every Shape

Cream of the Crop Short on length (in the sleeves, too) but long on style, this works as well with jeans as it does over a skirt.

Luxe Life A wide collar and defined waistline flatters a range of figures without compromising style.

Deconstruction Zone A basic camel coat becomes something cooler when it's spliced and tweaked.

{50s}

Trimming silhouettes with flare, not froth, are your fashion calling cards for both work and play

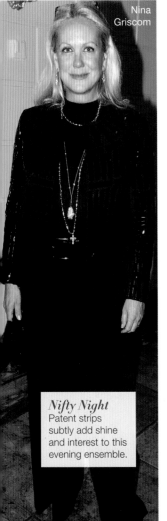

Nina Griscom

Nifty Night
Patent strips subtly add shine and interest to this evening ensemble.

• **Pump up the prints.** Too much frippery looks cluttered, bulky, and young, but you can turn heads with luscious floral prints and crisp geometrics instead.

• **3-D isn't just for the movies.** Texture and tone-on-tone (including black) can lend even the simplest and sparest jackets and coats depth while still keeping the overall effect clean and unfettered.

• **Don't forget to relax.** Women sometimes err too much on the side of dressy, ignoring their everyday sartorial needs. A casual well-worn, toss-on blazer or cropped warm woolen will do the trick.

• **It takes a little finesse.** Long gone are the days of chocking up a frayed hem or missing button as louche affectation. Keeping it together is the height of style.

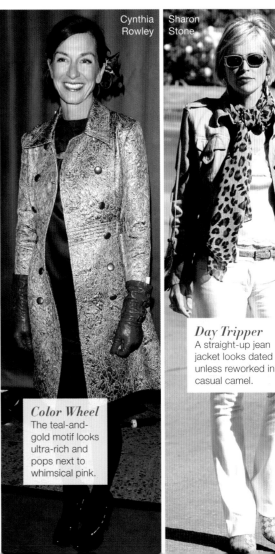

Cynthia Rowley

Sharon Stone

Day Tripper
A straight-up jean jacket looks dated unless reworked in casual camel.

Color Wheel
The teal-and-gold motif looks ultra-rich and pops next to whimsical pink.

Editors' Picks

Peacoat Peek
The sailor's staple is reborn with a 1960s-like collar and exaggerated proportion.

Bead Beat If you're going to pile on the beadwork, avoid an overpowering look by keeping it in the same color family.

Grape Crush At first glance, a simple coat. Look again, and notice the gracefully curved collar and elegant silhouette.

White Coat Let girlish effects give way to cool structural lines and contrast.

Great for Every Shape

Flower Power
A spray of perky buds is the pinnacle of dressing up like a lady.

Matrix Madame
Smart styling turns a sci-fi overcoat into a stunningly gorgeous evening piece.

Well-Worn Denim Cuff the sleeves of a denim blazer and you've got a casual new layer. Belt it for more shape.

{60s}

Sophistication reigns with a slew of long, lean coats and elegant jackets

• **An elongated car coat should be your go-to.** The extra bit of length for day gives you leaner proportions. Buttoned and belted it can even serve as a dress.

• **Keep it light.** Bulkier materials can add unwanted volume and clunky lines. Thankfully, even winter toppers come in lighter wools that will still keep the frost far away.

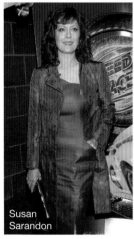

Susan Sarandon

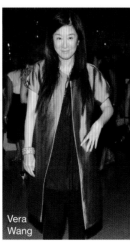

Vera Wang

Subtle Sheen
The mix of a blue floral against rich brown makes for a lovely evening outfit.

Haute Top
A zip- and button-free silk coat—this is one time you can go without closure.

{70+}

As grande dame, you can slip into a pleasing plethora of beautiful looks

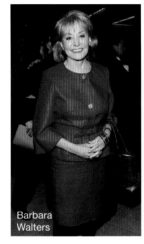

Barbara Walters

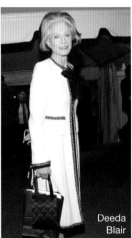

Deeda Blair

Hot Hues
Light up your face with a bright color that complements your undertones.

Ebony and Ivory
Black and white really do live together in perfect harmony.

• **Belted, but of course.** A quick and easy way to update a beloved old coat or jacket is by cinching it with a belt. Each one will bring new energy to your wardrobe.

• **Sometimes, it's just that simple.** In a world that's increasingly cluttered, a clean, fuss-free look is a refreshing and fashion-forward move, and one that's full of grace.

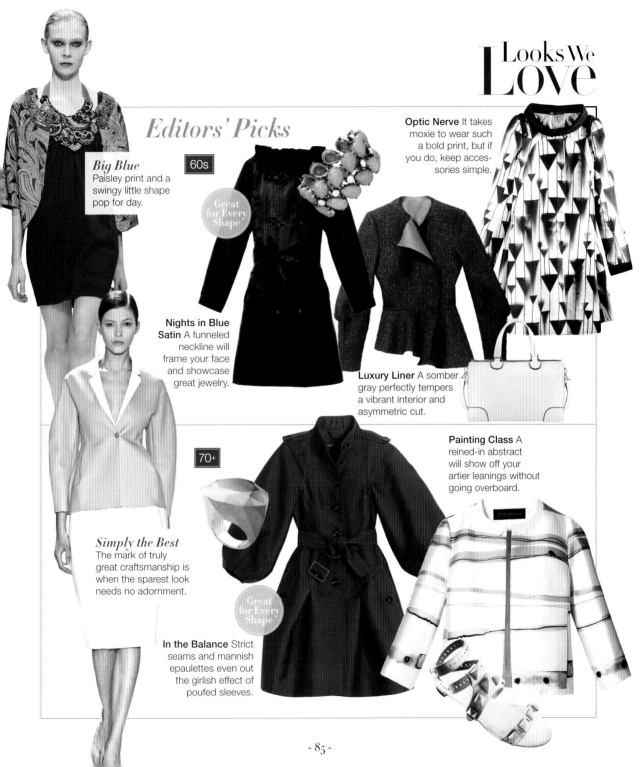

Editors' Picks

60s

Great for Every Shape

Big Blue
Paisley print and a swingy little shape pop for day.

Optic Nerve It takes moxie to wear such a bold print, but if you do, keep accessories simple.

Nights in Blue
Satin A funneled neckline will frame your face and showcase great jewelry.

Luxury Liner A somber gray perfectly tempers a vibrant interior and asymmetric cut.

70+

Painting Class A reined-in abstract will show off your artier leanings without going overboard.

Simply the Best
The mark of truly great craftsmanship is when the sparest look needs no adornment.

Great for Every Shape

In the Balance Strict seams and mannish epaulettes even out the girlish effect of poufed sleeves.

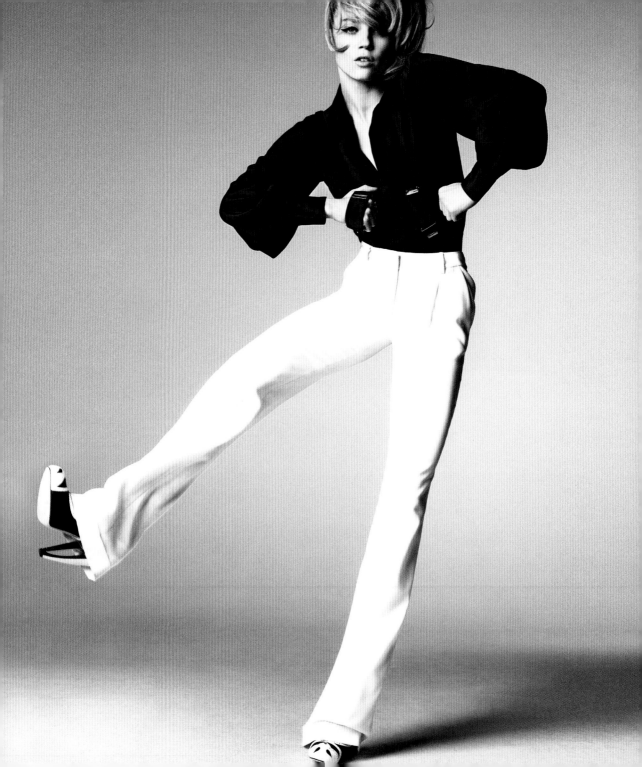

CHAPTER SIX

How to Wear It: Pants

Pants may seem like one of the harder separates to maneuver, but when you know what to look for in fit and style, stocking your closet with both the fun and the timeless is a breeze. Too curvy? Go for long and straight. Petite? Try high-waisted. Long and lanky? Pump up the volume

{ "Pants emit a very sexy, slightly masculine, wholly durable sensibility. They are reflective of the demeanor of a strong and stylish woman." —FRIDA GIANNINI }

{20s}

Take advantage of your "young enough to pull it off" status and explore the less traditional side of trousers

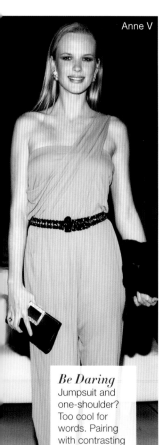

Anne V

• **Getting leggy can still be sophisticated.** There's life to explore beyond gym shorts and cutoffs. Even the mini-est come in tailored incarnations.

• **Make a statement.** As a rule, it's best to avoid anything that needs an instruction manual to get into. But in this decade, you can give tricky pants (pleats, poufs, jodhpurs, harems) a whirl.

• **Dapper is downtown cool.** A suit is more than the sum of its parts. The pants alone make terrific neutral separates. Pair with anything from sexy camis and edgy jewelry to buttoned-up shirts and baggy sweaters.

• **Long live leggings.** Whether they're considered hosiery or pants is beside the point. These comfy pieces make a great extra layer and come in ultra-stylish new ways.

Be Daring
Jumpsuit and one-shoulder? Too cool for words. Pairing with contrasting accessories only ups the ante.

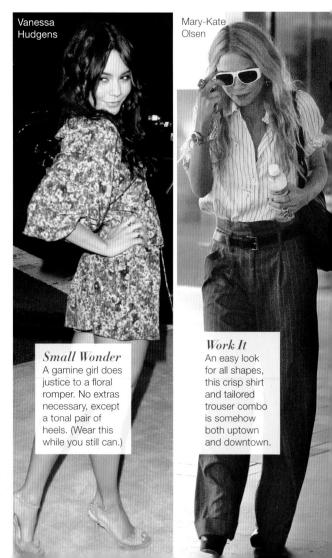

Vanessa Hudgens

Mary-Kate Olsen

Small Wonder
A gamine girl does justice to a floral romper. No extras necessary, except a tonal pair of heels. (Wear this while you still can.)

Work It
An easy look for all shapes, this crisp shirt and tailored trouser combo is somehow both uptown and downtown.

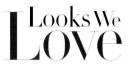
Editors' Picks

Tricks and Treats
The requisite cargo looks great in a silky, cropped silhouette for night.

In Tatters Whether by your hand or not, frays and tears make jeans look well loved.

Leather Leg
If you can get yourself into them (and peel yourself out), these are ultra stylish.

The Skinny
A stovepipe pant calls for exaggerated volume above.

Cargo Hold
Carpenter pants in camo green rank up there with the LBD in the wardrobe of staples.

Great for Every Shape

Easy Street
It's not exactly like wearing flannels out, but the right pajama bottom is great for day.

White Wow If you need a little more curve in your hips and derriere, a pouf and pleats will do the trick.

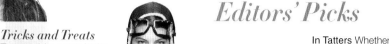

{30s}

Torn, tailored, skinny, baggy, short, long, dressed up, dressed down—pick a pant, any pant

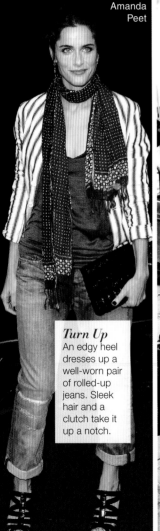

Amanda Peet

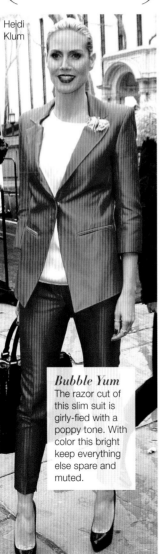

Heidi Klum

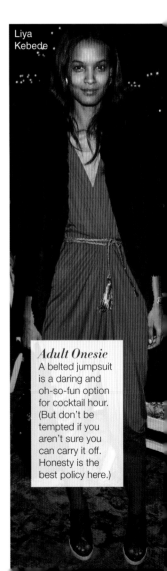

Liya Kebede

• **You can have both form and function.** There are plenty of work-appropriate slacks that still up your fashion quota. Try a pair of 1940s-era trousers or a cropped look with a crisp crease that's all business.

• **Try not to get into a rut with jeans.** If you know that a certain cut works well on you, by all means, stick to it— but also look for it in a different wash.

• **Think about pants for night.** They make a confident evening statement and open up a new world of accessorizing options.

• **You're still young— at heart and at dressing.** Some lengths may now read too young, but you can still pull off other more involved looks— like cuffed pants or a disco-diva jumpsuit in forgiving jersey.

Turn Up
An edgy heel dresses up a well-worn pair of rolled-up jeans. Sleek hair and a clutch take it up a notch.

Bubble Yum
The razor cut of this slim suit is girly-fied with a poppy tone. With color this bright keep everything else spare and muted.

Adult Onesie
A belted jumpsuit is a daring and oh-so-fun option for cocktail hour. (But don't be tempted if you aren't sure you can carry it off. Honesty is the best policy here.)

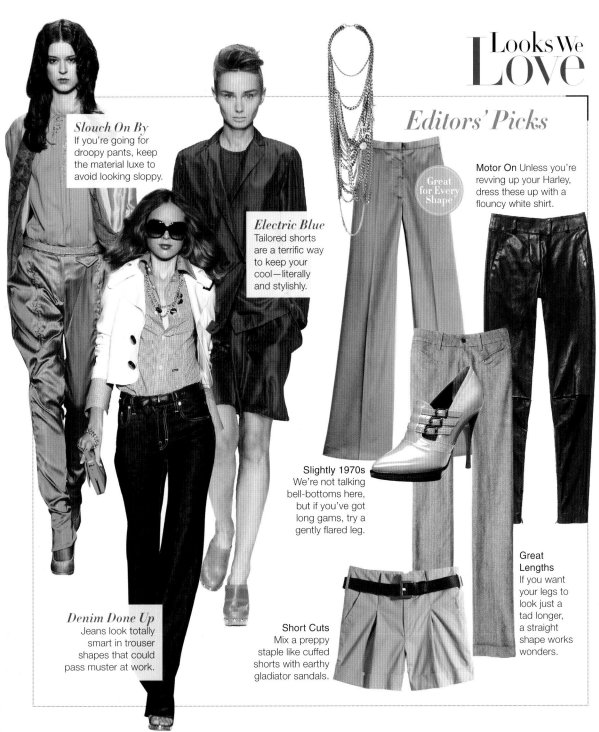

Looks We Love

Editors' Picks

Slouch On By
If you're going for droopy pants, keep the material luxe to avoid looking sloppy.

Electric Blue
Tailored shorts are a terrific way to keep your cool—literally and stylishly.

Great for Every Shape

Motor On Unless you're revving up your Harley, dress these up with a flouncy white shirt.

Slightly 1970s
We're not talking bell-bottoms here, but if you've got long gams, try a gently flared leg.

Denim Done Up
Jeans look totally smart in trouser shapes that could pass muster at work.

Short Cuts
Mix a preppy staple like cuffed shorts with earthy gladiator sandals.

Great Lengths
If you want your legs to look just a tad longer, a straight shape works wonders.

{4Os}

In or out of the office, trousers are an increasingly important element to dressing way up

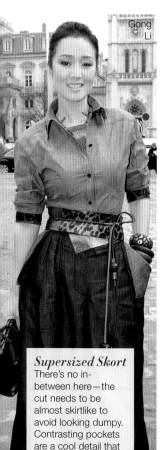

Gong Li

• **Annie Hall is an eternal fashion icon for good reason.** Right about now, working the iconic vest-and-men's-trousers look lends you a sexy, confident air.

• **Where's your tailor, Savile Row?** Maybe not, but tailoring every pant you buy to your figure (even jeans) is a top expert tip.

• **Cut from the finest cloth.** Pieces like trousers, which bear the brunt of multiple wearings, will last longer if they're made from quality materials.

• **A tux is a must.** Now subtly sexy is more appropriate than va-va-voom. A great man's suit in black is über-sexy. Tie optional.

• **Get glittering extras.** Even the most straight-forward pants look sharp with a touch of the shiny stuff—especially on shoes.

Supersized Skort
There's no in-between here—the cut needs to be almost skirtlike to avoid looking dumpy. Contrasting pockets are a cool detail that also create a slimming illusion.

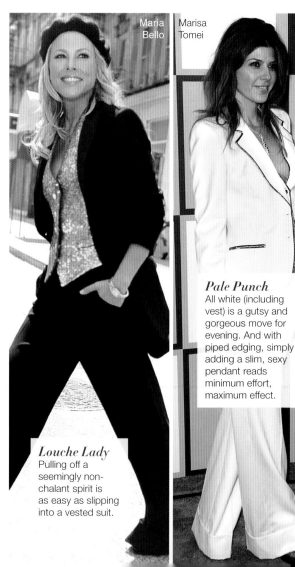

Maria Bello

Marisa Tomei

Pale Punch
All white (including vest) is a gutsy and gorgeous move for evening. And with piped edging, simply adding a slim, sexy pendant reads minimum effort, maximum effect.

Louche Lady
Pulling off a seemingly non-chalant spirit is as easy as slipping into a vested suit.

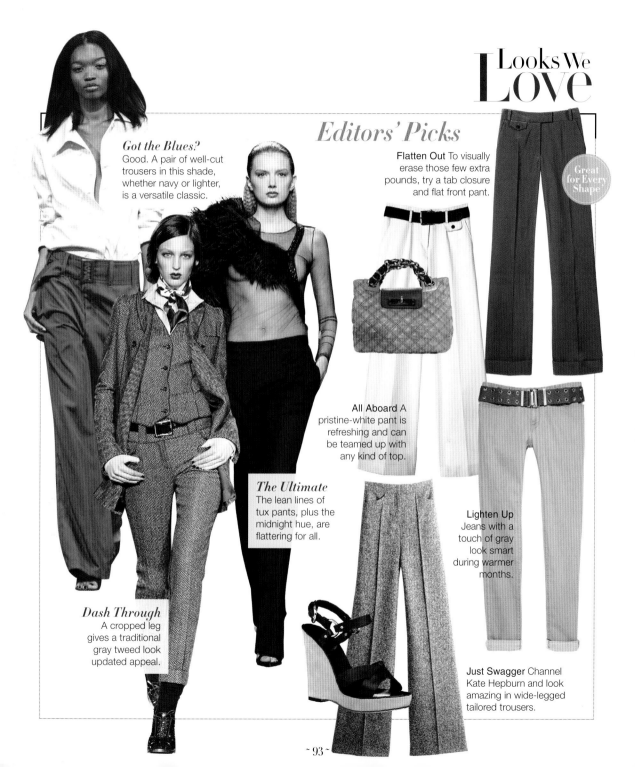

Got the Blues?
Good. A pair of well-cut trousers in this shade, whether navy or lighter, is a versatile classic.

Editors' Picks

Flatten Out To visually erase those few extra pounds, try a tab closure and flat front pant.

Great for Every Shape

All Aboard A pristine-white pant is refreshing and can be teamed up with any kind of top.

The Ultimate
The lean lines of tux pants, plus the midnight hue, are flattering for all.

Lighten Up
Jeans with a touch of gray look smart during warmer months.

Dash Through
A cropped leg gives a traditional gray tweed look updated appeal.

Just Swagger Channel Kate Hepburn and look amazing in wide-legged tailored trousers.

{50s}

Day or night, it's a good idea to mix color and shape for maximum styling versatility

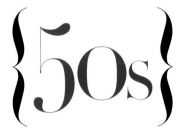

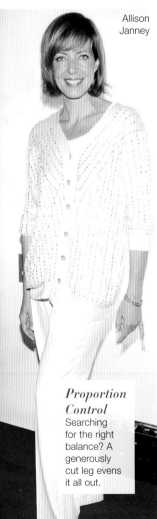

Allison Janney

Proportion Control
Searching for the right balance? A generously cut leg evens it all out.

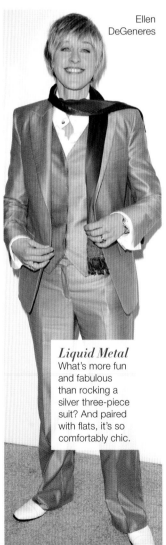

Ellen DeGeneres

Liquid Metal
What's more fun and fabulous than rocking a silver three-piece suit? And paired with flats, it's so comfortably chic.

• **Go with the flow.** It's OK to relax the strict tailoring rule for evening by donning a pair of pajama-like pants. Just don't let things get too loosey-goosey.

• **Stare at your feet.** Your pants and shoes are each other's closest allies. Do they look good together? When you're buying one, keep the other in mind.

• **From black to white and everywhere in between**. Even if you look best in only one or two styles of trouser, it needn't limit your options. You should try them in different colors.

• **To pleat or not to pleat? That is the eternal question**. If you're hippy, we advise against it, though you could *try* a pair in a super-super-relaxed fit.

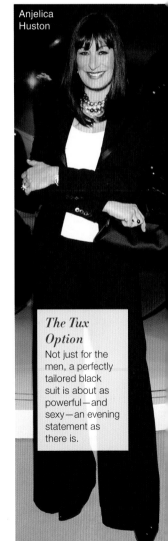

Anjelica Huston

The Tux Option
Not just for the men, a perfectly tailored black suit is about as powerful—and sexy—an evening statement as there is.

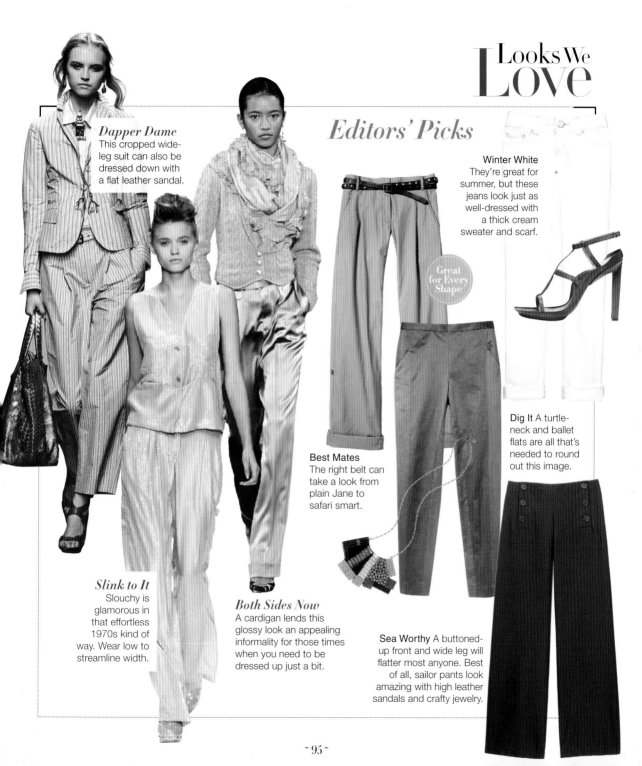

Looks We Love

Editors' Picks

Dapper Dame
This cropped wide-leg suit can also be dressed down with a flat leather sandal.

Winter White
They're great for summer, but these jeans look just as well-dressed with a thick cream sweater and scarf.

Great for Every Shape

Best Mates
The right belt can take a look from plain Jane to safari smart.

Dig It A turtleneck and ballet flats are all that's needed to round out this image.

Slink to It
Slouchy is glamorous in that effortless 1970s kind of way. Wear low to streamline width.

Both Sides Now
A cardigan lends this glossy look an appealing informality for those times when you need to be dressed up just a bit.

Sea Worthy A buttoned-up front and wide leg will flatter most anyone. Best of all, sailor pants look amazing with high leather sandals and crafty jewelry.

{6Os}

Keep in mind that basics and traditional styles are eternally classy

- **Forget the bells and whistles.** Modern sophistication is often defined by stripping away the details and letting impeccable finish and tailoring shine through.

- **Your pants are your support crew.** They provide the neutral backdrop on which to show off accessories, like red heels or a vintage coin belt.

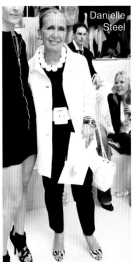

Danielle Steel

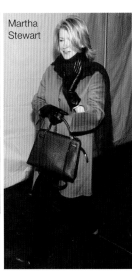

Martha Stewart

Opposites Attract
Black pants get a mod pick-me-up with vibrant contrasting mates.

City Chic
Keep a dark pair on hand for trips around town when you still want to look your best.

{7O+}

When you have the right trousers, you can toy with so many diverse styles

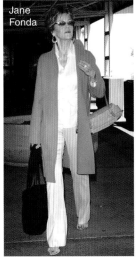

Jane Fonda

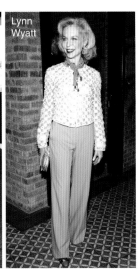

Lynn Wyatt

Jet Set
Wherever you go, so go your pants. Fabrics that wrinkle easily will slow you down.

In Neutral
If you buy just one, a classic gray (pale or charcoal) can carry any other color or motif.

- **Too many trousers?** No way. You can never really have enough of a good thing, especially if they slim and lengthen. Plus, you can top them with feminine frills or minimal pieces.

- **Slim and slimmer.** Skintight is definitely not an option, no matter what age you are, but body-skimming lines are always a sleek choice.

Editors' Picks

60s

Metal Works

White is a great back-drop for showcasing your favorite metallic accessories during the day.

Get in Line
The tuxedo stripe magically makes legs appear inches longer and slimmer.

Great for Every Shape

Country Girl
It's off to the manor when you pair a tony brown boot with a checked trouser.

70+

It All Adds Up A high waist (plus a platform) gives legs that go-on-for-miles effect we all dream of.

Great for Every Shape

Just Like PJs

Dress up comfortable, soft options with striking heels and belts.

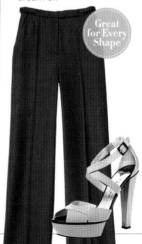

On Trend You can always interpret the runways to suit your style, like cuffing a silky loose number instead of jeans.

In Good Measure We mean literally. A cut that falls straight from the hips creates the most pleasing shape.

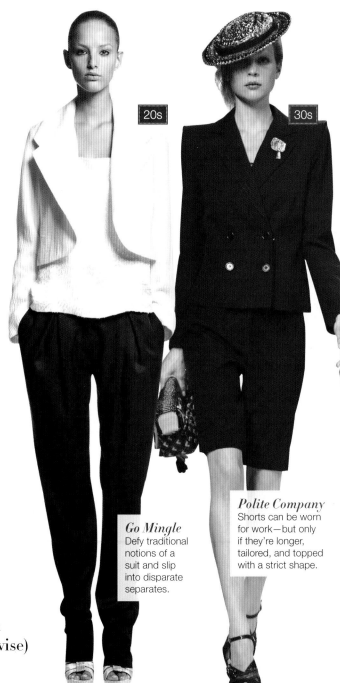

20s

30s

Pant Suits

It definitely isn't a man's world—it's one where anyone can rock a stylish jacket and pant (matching or otherwise)

Go Mingle
Defy traditional notions of a suit and slip into disparate separates.

Polite Company
Shorts can be worn for work—but only if they're longer, tailored, and topped with a strict shape.

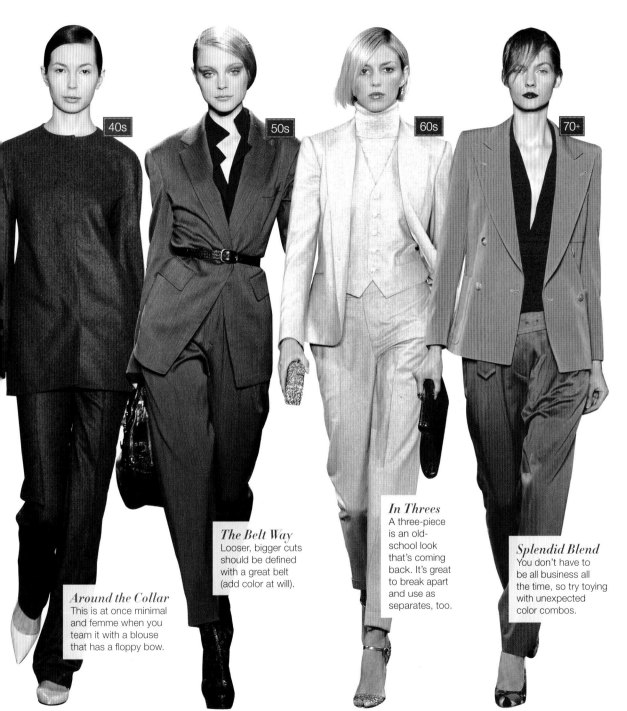

40s

50s

60s

70+

The Belt Way
Looser, bigger cuts
should be defined
with a great belt
(add color at will).

In Threes
A three-piece
is an old-
school look
that's coming
back. It's great
to break apart
and use as
separates, too.

Splendid Blend
You don't have to
be all business all
the time, so try toying
with unexpected
color combos.

Around the Collar
This is at once minimal
and femme when you
team it with a blouse
that has a floppy bow.

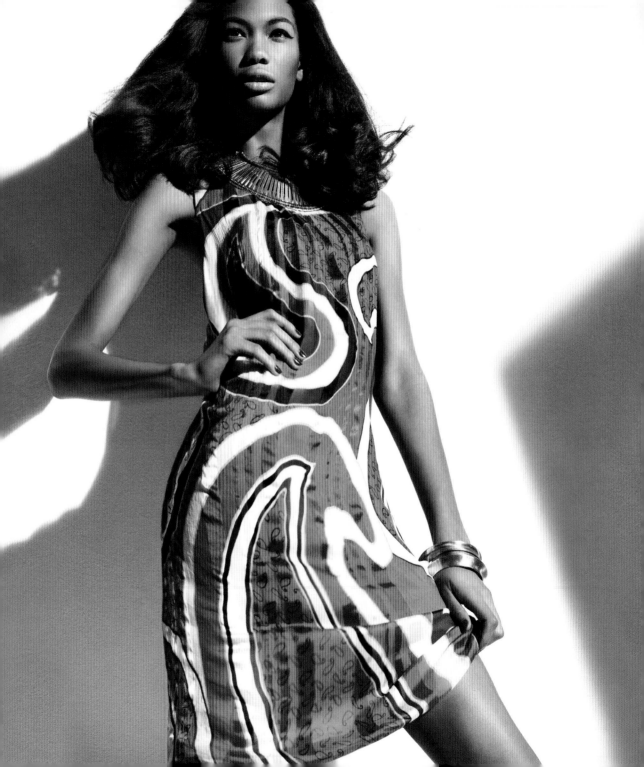

CHAPTER SEVEN

How to Wear It: Dresses

Sometimes just one piece is all you need—simply throw on a frock and go. But you can also use it as a building block for great styling and showing off your personality. A dress can be both alluringly feminine and confidently empowering at the same time

{ "If you have the right attitude and you wear the clothes in the right way, you have a natural sexiness." —STELLA MCCARTNEY }

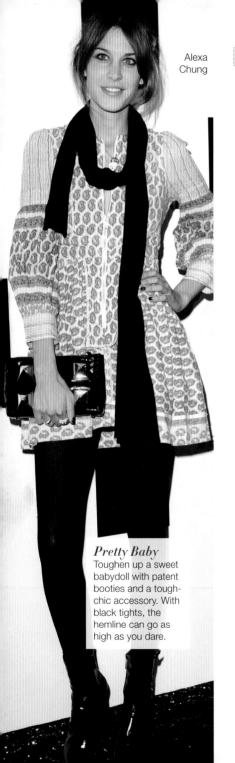

Alexa Chung

Pretty Baby
Toughen up a sweet babydoll with patent booties and a tough-chic accessory. With black tights, the hemline can go as high as you dare.

{ 20s }

Fill your closets with short, girly fare and edgy, experimental goods alike

• **It's OK not to commit**. You're still developing your style, and with such diverse offerings, the day dress is a perfect way to explore different fashion genres.

• **But it's OK to commit, too.** Plenty of women cultivate their vibe right out of their teens (if not during). And even if you subscribe to a certain beat, like minimal, layered louche, or boho, there is still a lot of experimenting to be done. There are many great ways within a particular style to work a dress.

• **Dressing the same piece up or down will smartly stretch your budget and mix up your look.** Switching shoes and throwing on a belt or chain can make a world of difference.

• **Make the most of this moment.** At some point, such youthful trappings as tons of frills, bows, and sugary-sweet prints won't look age-appropriate anymore. So indulge those leanings pronto.

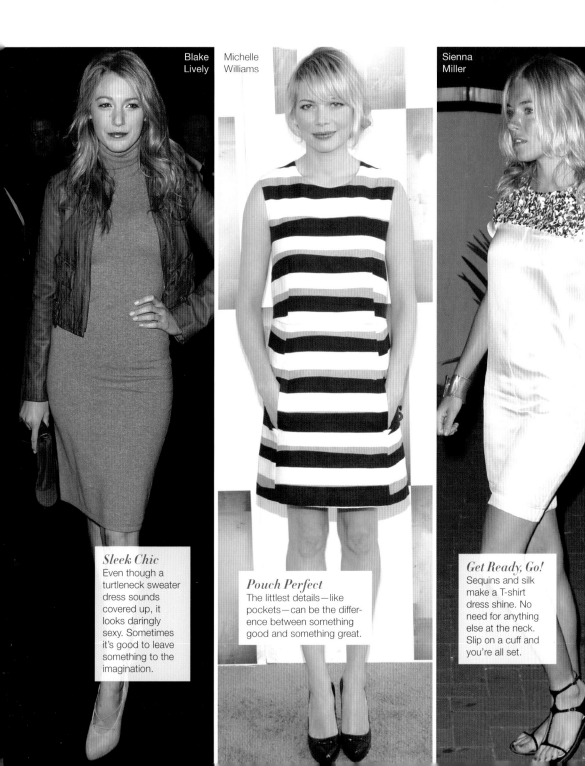

Blake
Lively

Michelle
Williams

Sienna
Miller

Sleek Chic
Even though a
turtleneck sweater
dress sounds
covered up, it
looks daringly
sexy. Sometimes
it's good to leave
something to the
imagination.

Pouch Perfect
The littlest details—like
pockets—can be the difference between something
good and something great.

Get Ready, Go!
Sequins and silk
make a T-shirt
dress shine. No
need for anything
else at the neck.
Slip on a cuff and
you're all set.

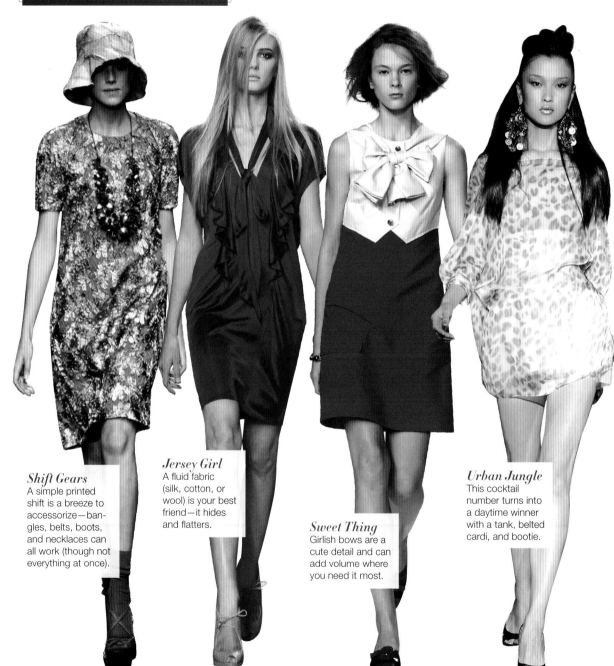

Shift Gears
A simple printed shift is a breeze to accessorize—bangles, belts, boots, and necklaces can all work (though not everything at once).

Jersey Girl
A fluid fabric (silk, cotton, or wool) is your best friend—it hides and flatters.

Sweet Thing
Girlish bows are a cute detail and can add volume where you need it most.

Urban Jungle
This cocktail number turns into a daytime winner with a tank, belted cardi, and bootie.

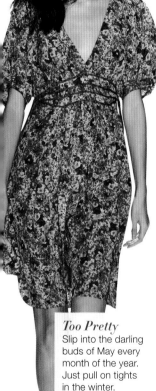

Looks We Love

Allow yourself free rein when it comes to picking dresses. Anything goes

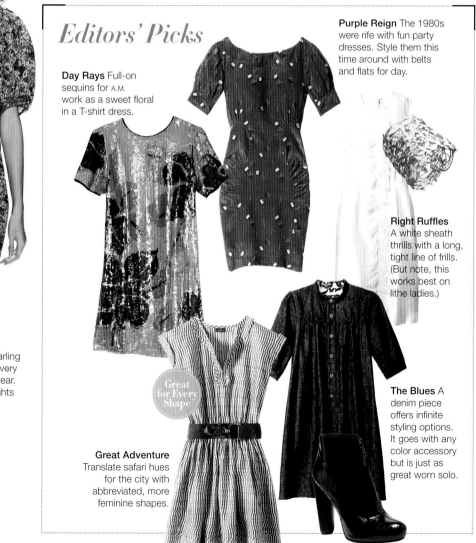

Editors' Picks

Day Rays Full-on sequins for A.M. work as a sweet floral in a T-shirt dress.

Purple Reign The 1980s were rife with fun party dresses. Style them this time around with belts and flats for day.

Right Ruffles A white sheath thrills with a long, tight line of frills. (But note, this works best on lithe ladies.)

Great for Every Shape

Great Adventure Translate safari hues for the city with abbreviated, more feminine shapes.

The Blues A denim piece offers infinite styling options. It goes with any color accessory but is just as great worn solo.

Too Pretty Slip into the darling buds of May every month of the year. Just pull on tights in the winter.

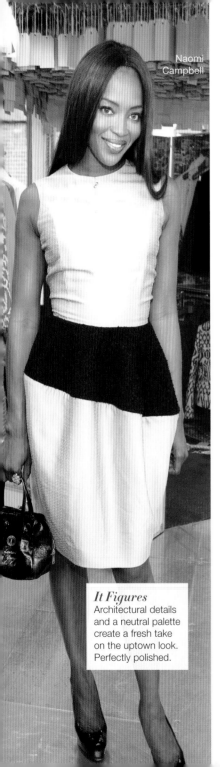

Naomi
Campbell

It Figures
Architectural details
and a neutral palette
create a fresh take
on the uptown look.
Perfectly polished.

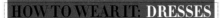

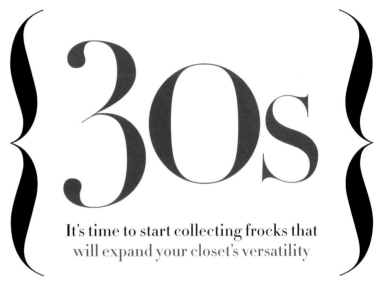

{ 3Os }

It's time to start collecting frocks that
will expand your closet's versatility

• **Raising the bar.** If you're going to go for a shorter hem (no higher than midthigh), cover up on top. Too much skin above and below isn't appropriate anywhere.

• **Fake it if you want to make it.** Not everyone is blessed with voluptuous dimensions. But creating curves is easy with a well-placed ruffle at the bust, hip, or even at the small of your back to accentuate your derriere.

• **Practice balance.** A cardinal rule is never to skew too far in one direction, like being so strictly minimal you only own black and gray shifts. It's hard to maintain and you'd miss out on the joy of injecting some hot pink into all that sobriety.

• **Watching the weather gets tedious.** Buy dresses that can go year-round with some smart styling.

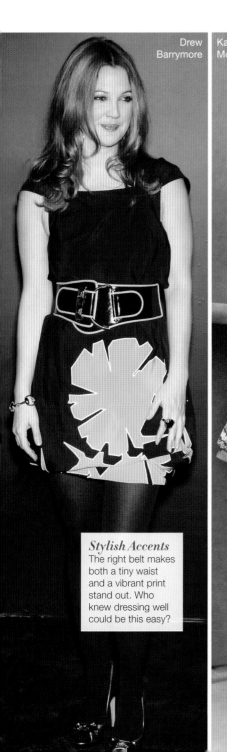

Drew
Barrymore

Stylish Accents
The right belt makes
both a tiny waist
and a vibrant print
stand out. Who
knew dressing well
could be this easy?

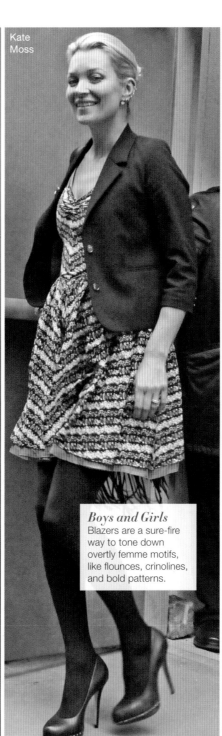

Kate
Moss

Boys and Girls
Blazers are a sure-fire
way to tone down
overtly femme motifs,
like flounces, crinolines,
and bold patterns.

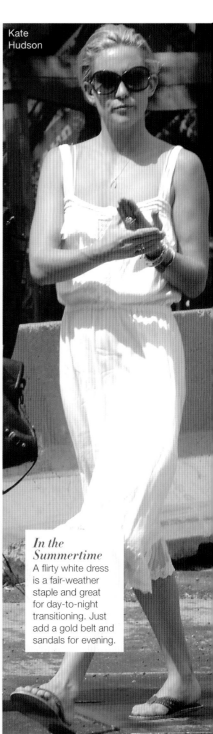

Kate
Hudson

In the Summertime
A flirty white dress
is a fair-weather
staple and great
for day-to-night
transitioning. Just
add a gold belt and
sandals for evening.

HOW TO WEAR IT: DRESSES

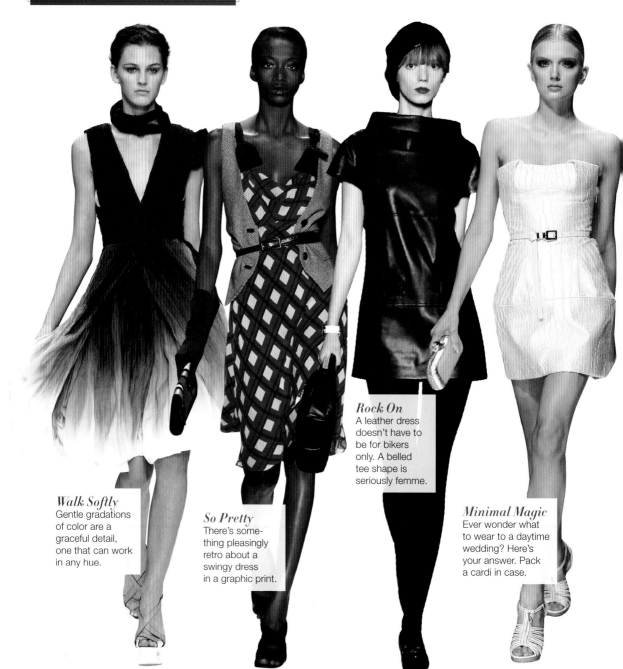

Walk Softly
Gentle gradations of color are a graceful detail, one that can work in any hue.

So Pretty
There's something pleasingly retro about a swingy dress in a graphic print.

Rock On
A leather dress doesn't have to be for bikers only. A belled tee shape is seriously femme.

Minimal Magic
Ever wonder what to wear to a daytime wedding? Here's your answer. Pack a cardi in case.

Looks We Love

Delve into the many wonders of ribbons, beads, ruches, pin tucks, and pleats

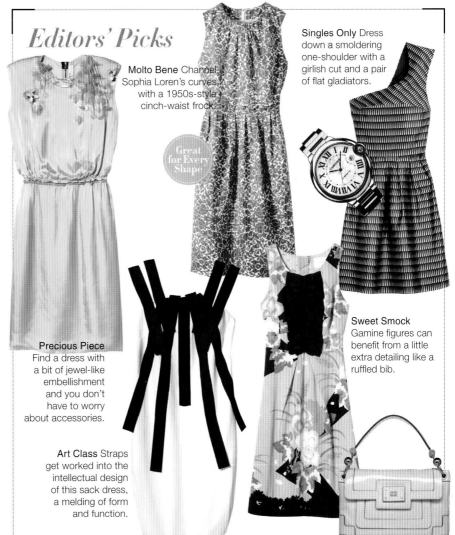

Editors' Picks

Molto Bene Channel Sophia Loren's curves with a 1950s-style cinch-waist frock.

Great for Every Shape

Singles Only Dress down a smoldering one-shoulder with a girlish cut and a pair of flat gladiators.

Sweet Smock Gamine figures can benefit from a little extra detailing like a ruffled bib.

Precious Piece Find a dress with a bit of jewel-like embellishment and you don't have to worry about accessories.

Art Class Straps get worked into the intellectual design of this sack dress, a melding of form and function.

Sacking Out
The simplest shape is also the simplest to transform with a belt, a scarf, or a high shoe.

{40s}

Dresses anchor your entire wardrobe, from simple shifts to decorated numbers

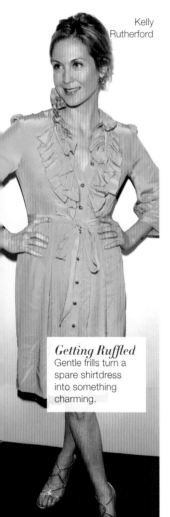

Kelly Rutherford

Getting Ruffled
Gentle frills turn a spare shirtdress into something charming.

• **What's your definition?** A shapeless frock does nothing for an hourglass or hippy figure. A cinched waist will prettily outline your curves and highlight your smallest part. If you absolutely love a particular sack dress, belt it.

• **History repeats itself.** The empire waist has been around for centuries because it flatters nearly everyone. It brings the attention to your décolletage but gives you breathing room elsewhere.

• **Going deep.** A V-neck instantly adds a few inches to your height. It's also a great stage for a bold choker or necklace.

• **Get the details.** Don't play it so safe your wardrobe is full of solids. Prints, patterns, pleats, and ruching are all pretty add-ons.

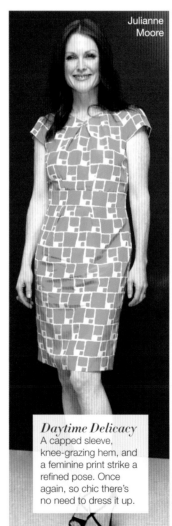

Julianne Moore

Daytime Delicacy
A capped sleeve, knee-grazing hem, and a feminine print strike a refined pose. Once again, so chic there's no need to dress it up.

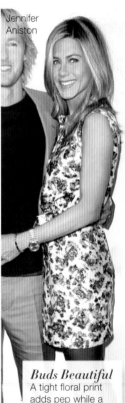

Jennifer Aniston

Buds Beautiful
A tight floral print adds pep while a cinched waist and shorter hem look modern.

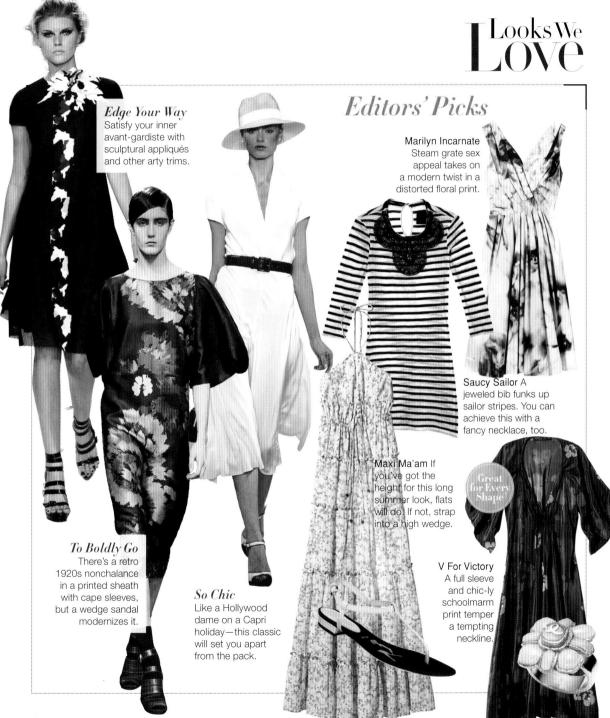

Editors' Picks

Edge Your Way
Satisfy your inner avant-gardiste with sculptural appliqués and other arty trims.

Marilyn Incarnate
Steam grate sex appeal takes on a modern twist in a distorted floral print.

Saucy Sailor A jeweled bib funks up sailor stripes. You can achieve this with a fancy necklace, too.

To Boldly Go
There's a retro 1920s nonchalance in a printed sheath with cape sleeves, but a wedge sandal modernizes it.

So Chic
Like a Hollywood dame on a Capri holiday—this classic will set you apart from the pack.

Maxi Ma'am If you've got the height for this long summer look, flats will do. If not, strap into a high wedge.

Great for Every Shape!

V For Victory
A full sleeve and chic-ly schoolmarm print temper a tempting neckline.

{ 50s }

The right fabrics and nipped-in silhouettes will keep you looking sensational and sophisticated

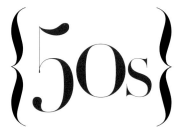

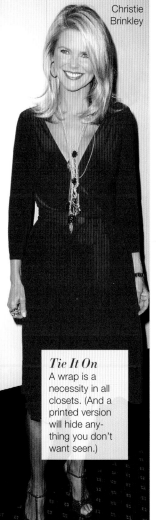

Christie Brinkley

Tie It On
A wrap is a necessity in all closets. (And a printed version will hide anything you don't want seen.)

• **What about silk for the office?** You have the gravitas to pull off a shinier material for day without looking like your fashion clock is fast. Just throw on a flat or chunky leather belt and sandal to complete the picture.

• **Oh, grow up. Prints, we mean.** If you're not sure whether or not a pattern is a little too young for you, some clever styling—a belted cardigan, double-stranded pearls, a large cuff—will age it appropriately.

• **Staying faithful (but occasionally straying).** Do you have favorite designers who season after season do right by you? That's fine, but it's worth flirting with new names sometimes.

• **All in one.** Wearing a solid hue, like a bright pink or gunmetal gray, can be as powerful as a print.

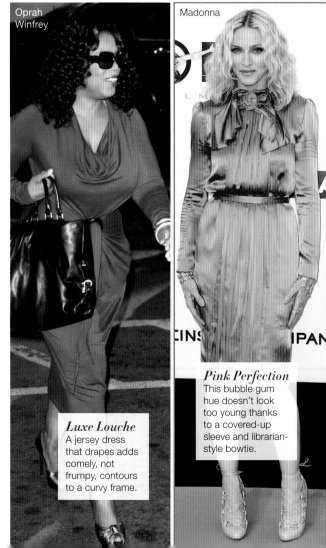

Oprah Winfrey

Madonna

Luxe Louche
A jersey dress that drapes adds comely, not frumpy, contours to a curvy frame.

Pink Perfection
This bubble gum hue doesn't look too young thanks to a covered-up sleeve and librarian-style bowtie.

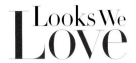

Print of Paradise
For the right occasion
(a wedding, for instance),
a louder print will win
you cheers, not jeers.

Editors' Picks

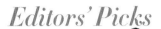

No Jewels Necessary
Avoid overaccessorizing a
printed frock that already
has an adorned neckline.
Go for a great ring instead.

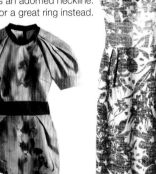

Equaling Out Don't
forget proportion. Here,
a slimmer skirt anchors
puffy shoulders.

In the Sack It's a
shape that's everywhere.
If you're slender, don
as is. If not, a belt will
add definition.

Great
for Every
Shape

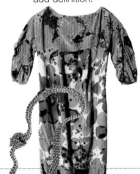

**Mercury
Rising**
Far from being
dull, gray is
increasingly a
go-to neutral
that can carry
any other color.

**Suddenly Last
Summer**
Lacy white, slightly off
the shoulder, belted
and flared—the closest
thing to a perfect
summer frock.

Plaid Tidings A
demonstrative graphic
and tight draping at
the hips will give you
all the right curves.

{6os}

Effortless dressing (and dresses) are the secret to keeping chic year-round

• **Being high-maintenance is a good thing.** And by that, we mean keeping up appointments with your tailor. Nipping a waist in or hemming an inch or two doesn't cost that much, and it'll be worth it when you get greater use out of a dress.

• **Keep it simple.** When in doubt—or if you're in a hurry—a plain sheath or shirtdress with a great shoe and belt is all you need.

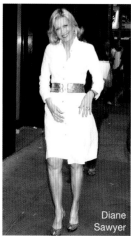

Diane Sawyer

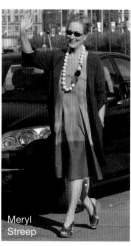

Meryl Streep

Gold Goddess
A wide metallic belt, echoed in the shoe, jazzes up an otherwise strict shirtdress.

The Eclectic
That easy-to-wear sack is destined to shine with bold, earthy necklaces and heels.

{7o+}

Your closet is so well stocked, now you can play with a different look every day

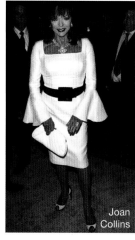

Joan Collins

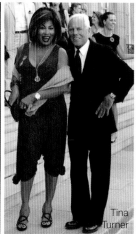

Tina Turner

Mod Maven
Contrasting colors pack a powerful visual punch. So do fancy sleeves.

Simply the Best
Cover up a daring show of skin with a wrap and a significantly sized pendant.

• **You know what we said about tailors?** They can also give new life to an old favorite. Take that 1970s-era caftan you just can't let go of: With a substantial nip and tuck, it can be a fab new sundress. It's a chic and economical way to recycle beloved pieces.

• **Match made in heaven.** Certain dresses are designed to be worn with stellar necklaces. Again, it's a good way to keep refreshing what's already in your closet.

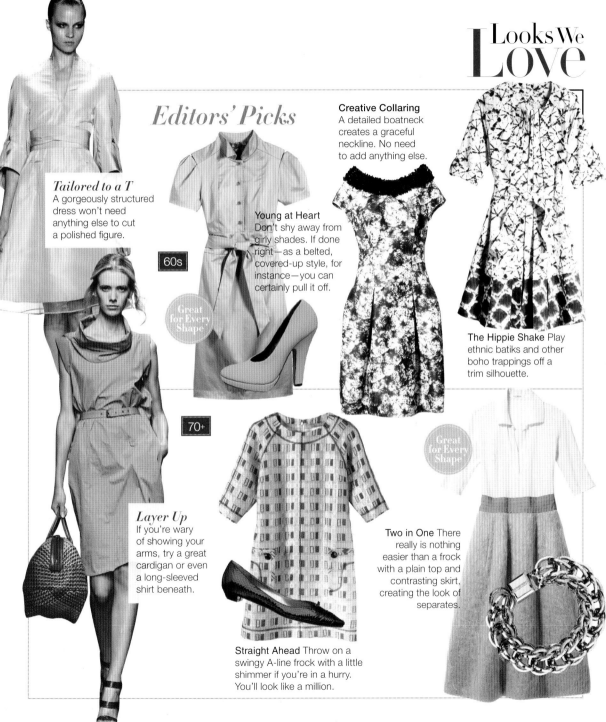

Editors' Picks

Tailored to a T
A gorgeously structured
dress won't need
anything else to cut
a polished figure.

60s

Great
for Every
Shape

Young at Heart
Don't shy away from
girly shades. If done
right—as a belted,
covered-up style, for
instance—you can
certainly pull it off.

Creative Collaring
A detailed boatneck
creates a graceful
neckline. No need
to add anything else.

The Hippie Shake Play
ethnic batiks and other
boho trappings off a
trim silhouette.

70+

Layer Up
If you're wary
of showing your
arms, try a great
cardigan or even
a long-sleeved
shirt beneath.

Straight Ahead Throw on a
swingy A-line frock with a little
shimmer if you're in a hurry.
You'll look like a million.

Two in One There
really is nothing
easier than a frock
with a plain top and
contrasting skirt,
creating the look of
separates.

Great
for Every
Shape

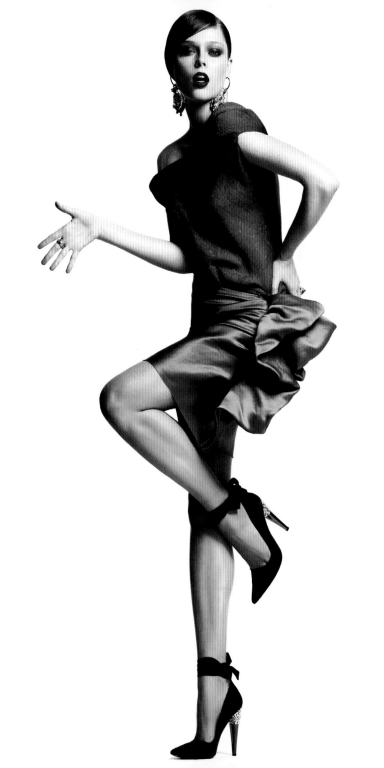

CHAPTER EIGHT

How to Wear It: Evening

As little girls, we dreamt of princess gowns and attending the ball. In reality, our dressing-up needs are more diverse (Cinderella never did cocktail) and a big pouf just isn't enough. This is when you should be wearing out-of-the-ordinary pieces, taking risks (within reason), and letting your spirit shine through

{ "You want an evening dress for many years, something that you can bring out again and again."—GEORGINA CHAPMAN }

{20s}

Girls just want to have fun. So right now you should play with the sexier, flirtier side of the night

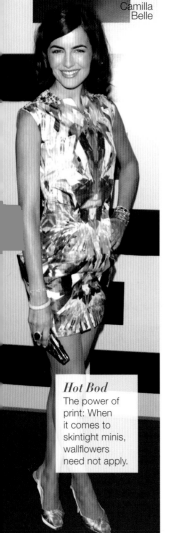

Camilla Belle

Hot Bod
The power of print: When it comes to skintight minis, wallflowers need not apply.

• **How tight is too tight?** If you're courageous enough and you've got the figure to pull it off, by all means go ahead. You know your own body shape.

• **Equal parts leg and heel is an equation to remember.** If you're going to show off your gams, a higher heel (preferably a thin one) will make them look longer and leaner.

• **Winning gold (and silver, bronze, and copper).** Metallics are a no-brainer for evening events, adding some flashy dash to the after-hours festivities.

• **Stunningly soigné is always on trend for events.** You can pull it all together in an instant by slipping into a timeless little black dress, a thin high heel, and just one piece of extraordinary costume jewelry.

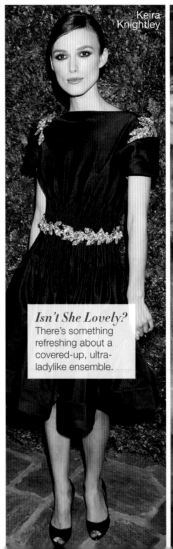

Keira Knightley

Isn't She Lovely?
There's something refreshing about a covered-up, ultra-ladylike ensemble.

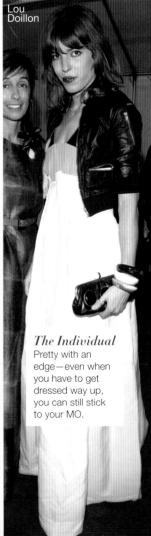

Lou Doillon

The Individual
Pretty with an edge—even when you have to get dressed way up, you can still stick to your MO.

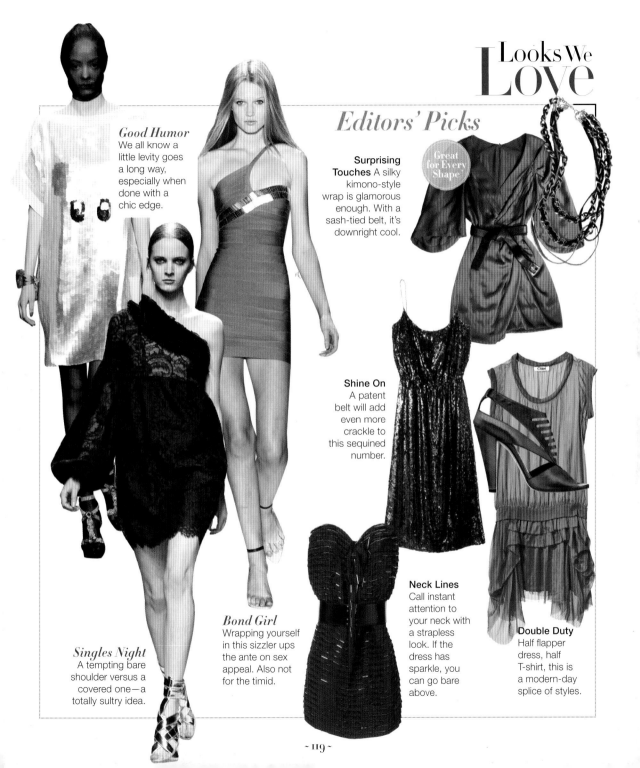

Editors' Picks

Good Humor We all know a little levity goes a long way, especially when done with a chic edge.

Surprising Touches A silky kimono-style wrap is glamorous enough. With a sash-tied belt, it's downright cool.

Great for Every Shape

Shine On A patent belt will add even more crackle to this sequined number.

Singles Night A tempting bare shoulder versus a covered one—a totally sultry idea.

Bond Girl Wrapping yourself in this sizzler ups the ante on sex appeal. Also not for the timid.

Neck Lines Call instant attention to your neck with a strapless look. If the dress has sparkle, you can go bare above.

Double Duty Half flapper dress, half T-shirt, this is a modern-day splice of styles.

{3os}

Evening is an especially thrilling time when beads, sequins, and jewels are involved

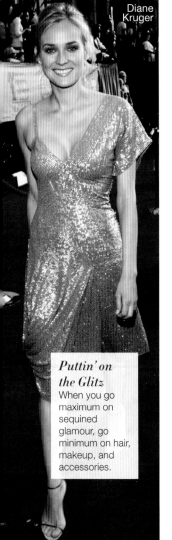

Diane Kruger

Puttin' on the Glitz
When you go maximum on sequined glamour, go minimum on hair, makeup, and accessories.

• **Go long.** Short and sexy or long and ballgown-y don't have to be your only two options. In this decade you can mix it *all* up, so what about trying a slim or fluid floor-grazer?

• **Go goddess.** Drapes and ruches create tempting curves when you need to add them— and accentuate the ones you've already got.

• **Go glam.** Don't shy away from the glitzy stuff. It can be done subtly, too, in darker hues and covered-up, body-skimming silhouettes.

• **Know your fashion geometry.** Asymmetry works as architectural details on the sleeve or neckline. But for hems, steer clear of overly obvious high-low lengths.

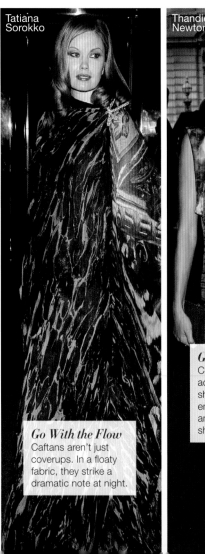

Tatiana Sorokko

Go With the Flow
Caftans aren't just coverups. In a floaty fabric, they strike a dramatic note at night.

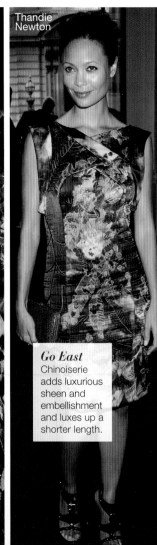

Thandie Newton

Go East
Chinoiserie adds luxurious sheen and embellishment and luxes up a shorter length.

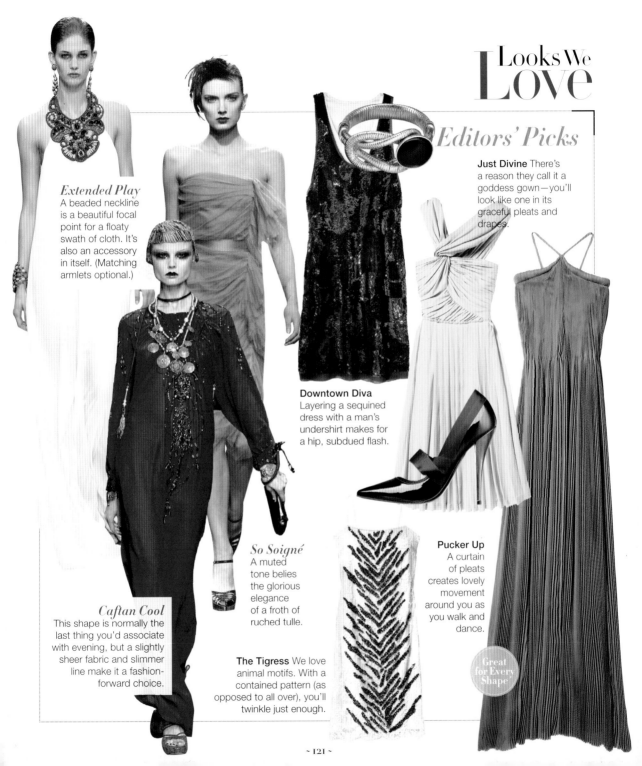

Editors' Picks

Extended Play
A beaded neckline is a beautiful focal point for a floaty swath of cloth. It's also an accessory in itself. (Matching armlets optional.)

Just Divine There's a reason they call it a goddess gown—you'll look like one in its graceful pleats and drapes.

Downtown Diva Layering a sequined dress with a man's undershirt makes for a hip, subdued flash.

So Soigné
A muted tone belies the glorious elegance of a froth of ruched tulle.

Caftan Cool
This shape is normally the last thing you'd associate with evening, but a slightly sheer fabric and slimmer line make it a fashion-forward choice.

The Tigress We love animal motifs. With a contained pattern (as opposed to all over), you'll twinkle just enough.

Pucker Up A curtain of pleats creates lovely movement around you as you walk and dance.

Great for Every Shape

{40s}

Turning up the shine and building on classics you've accrued in your closet is a sure-fire evening approach

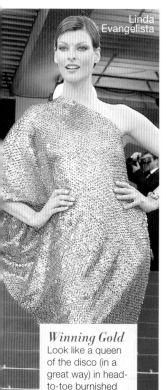

Linda Evangelista

Winning Gold
Look like a queen of the disco (in a great way) in head-to-toe burnished sparkles. Not for the faint-hearted.

- **Less is really more.** You've heard it before, but it bears repeating. It's sophisticated to let your gown outline your figure and showcase your confidence.

- **But more is fun, too.** Who doesn't like sequins and paillettes? Just remember the fashion fundamentals: If your dress is on the busier side, tone down your accessories.

- **Reining it all in.** A long frock doesn't need to take on ballgown dimensions. Keeping it slimmer is more modern.

- **Baring all.** The first lady has proved that if you've got toned arms, you can show them off. If not, a shawl will do beautifully.

- **When in doubt, accessorize.** Piling up long chains or cuffs to a day fare-thee-well can make it just right for night.

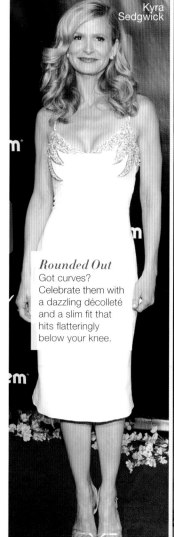

Kyra Sedgwick

Rounded Out
Got curves? Celebrate them with a dazzling décolleté and a slim fit that hits flatteringly below your knee.

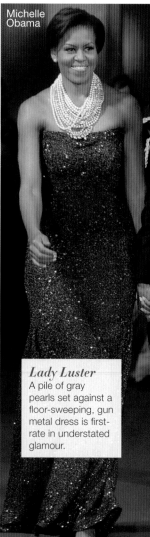

Michelle Obama

Lady Luster
A pile of gray pearls set against a floor-sweeping, gun metal dress is first-rate in understated glamour.

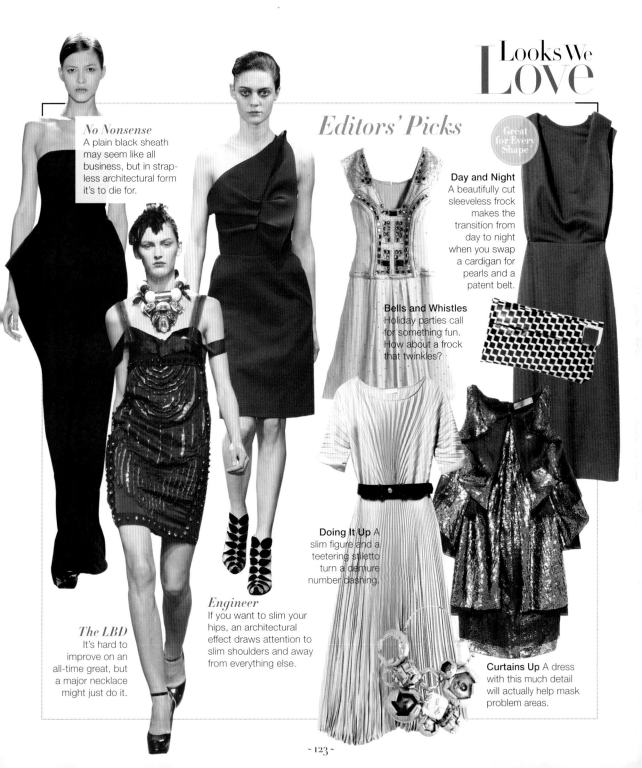

No Nonsense
A plain black sheath may seem like all business, but in strapless architectural form it's to die for.

Editors' Picks

Great
for Every
Shape

Day and Night
A beautifully cut sleeveless frock makes the transition from day to night when you swap a cardigan for pearls and a patent belt.

Bells and Whistles
Holiday parties call for something fun. How about a frock that twinkles?

Doing It Up A slim figure and a teetering stiletto turn a demure number dashing.

Engineer
If you want to slim your hips, an architectural effect draws attention to slim shoulders and away from everything else.

The LBD
It's hard to improve on an all-time great, but a major necklace might just do it.

Curtains Up A dress with this much detail will actually help mask problem areas.

{ 50s }

There's plenty of room for major declarations of style, from the simple to more unusual suspects

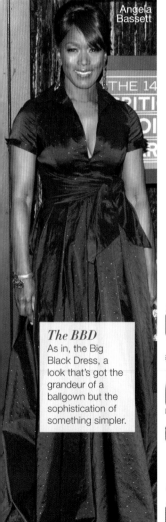

Angela Bassett

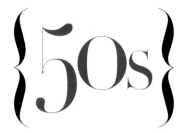

Trudie Styler

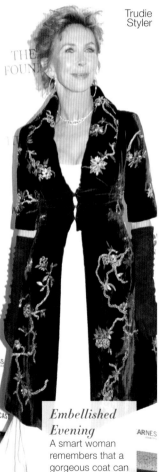

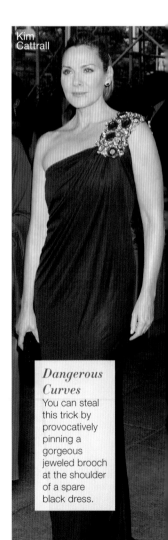

Kim Cattrall

• **Get excited about getting dressed.** After dark doesn't need to be a frustrating time to wriggle into pantyhose (go bare!) and uncomfortable girdles (not needed if you have the right fit). Approach it like an exciting break from the things you usually wear.

• **What a difference.** People generally view evening as a time to sex things up. Not always. It's more a moment to do something out of the ordinary, to shake things up and live a little. Pull out those far-out pieces you've been dying to wear but haven't had the nerve to.

• **What lengths will you go to?** There are no hard-and-fast rules on hem height for evening. The only one you should follow is what most flatters you.

The BBD
As in, the Big Black Dress, a look that's got the grandeur of a ballgown but the sophistication of something simpler.

Embellished Evening
A smart woman remembers that a gorgeous coat can be a scene stealer and intrinsic to an entire look.

Dangerous Curves
You can steal this trick by provocatively pinning a gorgeous jeweled brooch at the shoulder of a spare black dress.

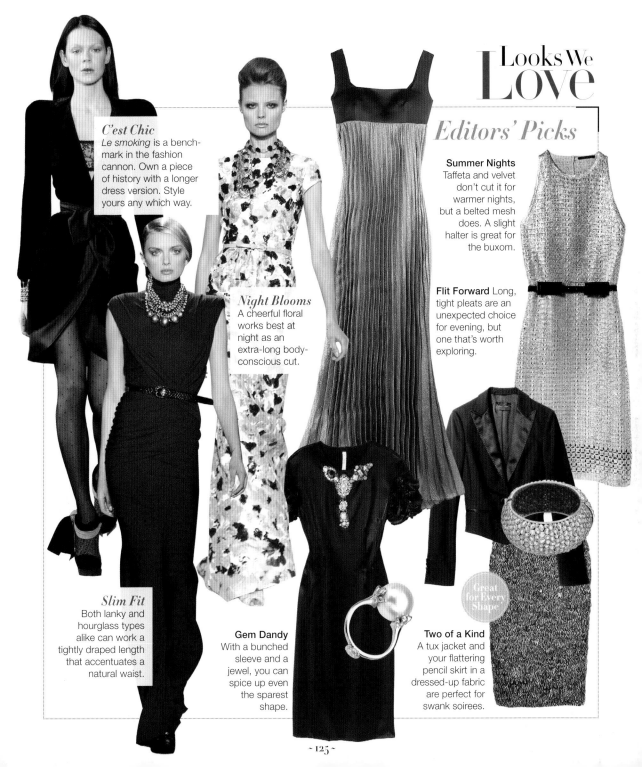

Looks We Love

Editors' Picks

C'est Chic
Le smoking is a benchmark in the fashion cannon. Own a piece of history with a longer dress version. Style yours any which way.

Summer Nights
Taffeta and velvet don't cut it for warmer nights, but a belted mesh does. A slight halter is great for the buxom.

Night Blooms
A cheerful floral works best at night as an extra-long body-conscious cut.

Flit Forward Long, tight pleats are an unexpected choice for evening, but one that's worth exploring.

Slim Fit
Both lanky and hourglass types alike can work a tightly draped length that accentuates a natural waist.

Gem Dandy
With a bunched sleeve and a jewel, you can spice up even the sparest shape.

Great for Every Shape

Two of a Kind
A tux jacket and your flattering pencil skirt in a dressed-up fabric are perfect for swank soirees.

{6Os}

Don't restrict yourself to shapeless frocks—it's all about fit and contour

• **Think outside your closet.** Evening is a good time to explore your adventurous side. If you normally play it safe, try different colors, prints, and textures.

• **Show a little skin.** That's right, the curve of a collar, a delicate wrist or ankle—there are less obvious ways to bare it.

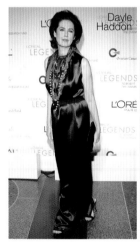

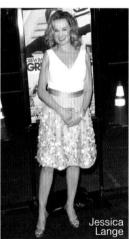

Jessica Lange

Liquid Languor
When broken down, it's really simple: long, long dress, belt, big necklace.

The Great Divide
If you look better in separates, choose a dress that mimics them.

{7O+}

Be the grande dame in the splendid looks others can only dream of

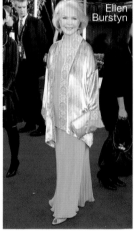

Ellen Burstyn

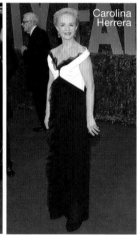

Carolina Herrera

Boudoir Bound
A silken bed jacket is the ultimate symbol of effortless style and total confidence.

Neck Lace
These slightly off-the-shoulder sleeves frame your décolletage and face.

• **A loose look doesn't have to be sloppy.** The right materials—like a chinoiserie silk—make the end result more languid and luxurious than anything else.

• **The finer points count for a lot,** like dangling earrings, beaded shoes, a noteworthy minaudière—and every hair in place.

• **Cover-ups optional.** If you're not crazy about your arms, grab an embellished shawl.

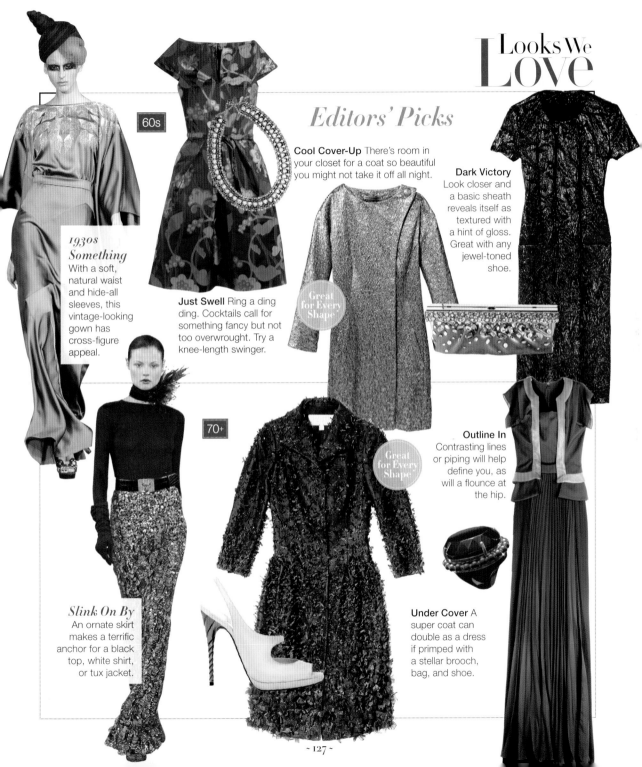

60s

Editors' Picks

Cool Cover-Up There's room in your closet for a coat so beautiful you might not take it off all night.

Dark Victory Look closer and a basic sheath reveals itself as textured with a hint of gloss. Great with any jewel-toned shoe.

1930s Something With a soft, natural waist and hide-all sleeves, this vintage-looking gown has cross-figure appeal.

Just Swell Ring a ding ding. Cocktails call for something fancy but not too overwrought. Try a knee-length swinger.

Great for Every Shape

70+

Great for Every Shape

Outline In Contrasting lines or piping will help define you, as will a flounce at the hip.

Slink On By An ornate skirt makes a terrific anchor for a black top, white shirt, or tux jacket.

Under Cover A super coat can double as a dress if primped with a stellar brooch, bag, and shoe.

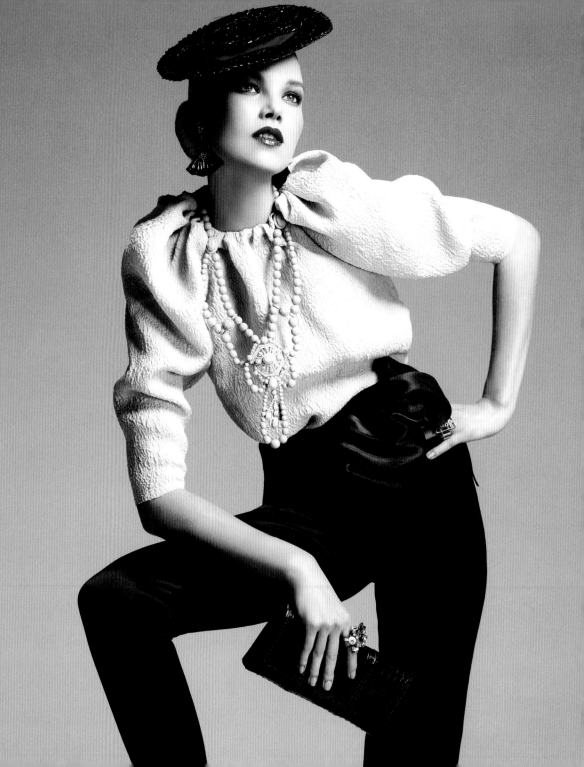

CHAPTER NINE

Best Extras

Accessories are democracy in action. No matter your age, shape, or size, you can humor any whim with shoes, bags, scarves, belts, and jewels. They have the ability to transform your look drastically and with minimal effort. And the smartest buys will last you a lifetime

{ "Like most girls, I understood at an early age that shoes are magic vessels." —REBECCA MILLER }

Ashley
Olsen

{20s}

Shoes

Your footwear speaks volumes about your personality:
rocker, glamour-puss, tough girl, hipster, hippie chic

• **Start with the five basics:** flat, leather sandal, boot, dress pump, and fun attention-grabber (sort of like dessert and totally your choice).

• **You might have to learn to walk all over again.** There's nothing more cringe inducing than watching a woman tottering in a precarious heel. Before you step out in those five-and-a-half-inch killers, practice so you can stride with confidence. If you're still off balance with a higher heel, most cobblers can shave a little off without compromising structure. (And if you really can't walk in them, don't waste your cash.)

• **Once you've got the essentials, let loose.** If there's something you especially love, like hot colors and bows for instance, shoes are a fun way to indulge the passion. A satin bubblegum pump with a floppy knot makes sense for evening, no?

• **How many is too many?** As easy as it would be to reenergize the world's economy by buying shoes alone, a little discipline is in order. Selecting what you will need and get a lot of use out of is the kind of responsible budget-balancing that will leave you with extra spending money at the end of the year. Then you can really have some fun.

True Blue
Sometimes all you need to complete the look is a bright strappy sandal.

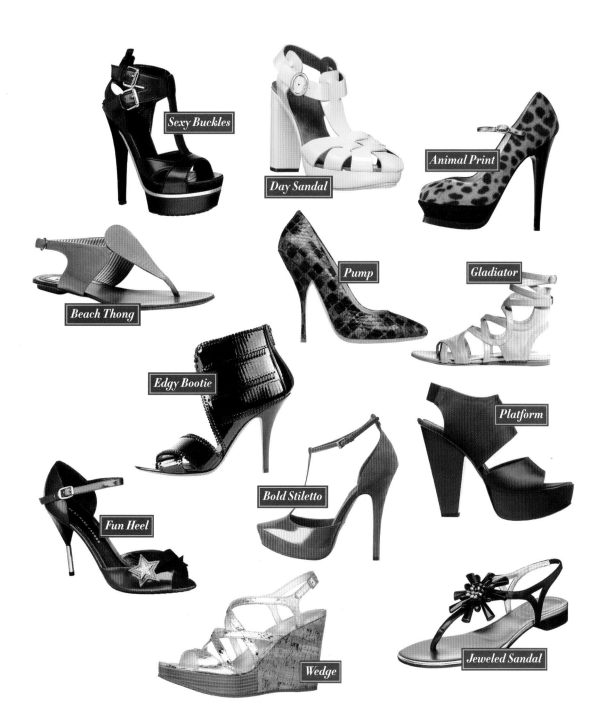

Sexy Buckles

Day Sandal

Animal Print

Beach Thong

Pump

Gladiator

Edgy Bootie

Platform

Fun Heel

Bold Stiletto

Wedge

Jeweled Sandal

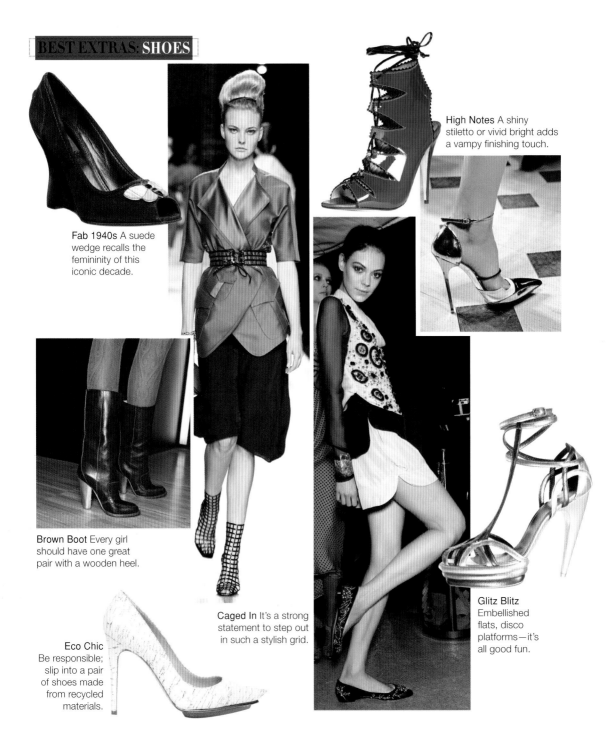

High Notes A shiny
stiletto or vivid bright adds
a vampy finishing touch.

Fab 1940s A suede
wedge recalls the
femininity of this
iconic decade.

Brown Boot Every girl
should have one great
pair with a wooden heel.

Caged In It's a strong
statement to step out
in such a stylish grid.

Glitz Blitz
Embellished
flats, disco
platforms—it's
all good fun.

Eco Chic
Be responsible;
slip into a pair
of shoes made
from recycled
materials.

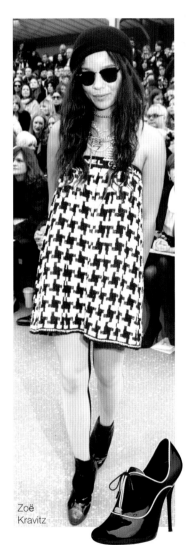

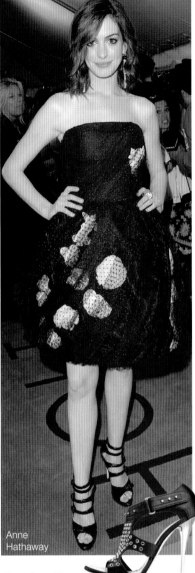

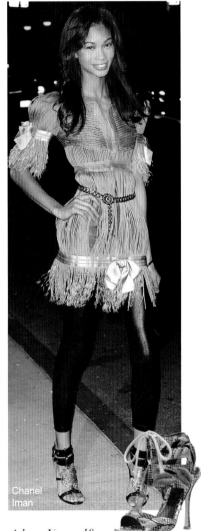

Anne
Hathaway

Zoë
Kravitz

Chanel
Iman

Toughen Up
Balance an overtly girlish
ensemble with a heel that
has a harder edge.

Bootie-Licious
A little black kid boot
can go both ways—
ladylike or rocker.

Adorn Yourself
Sparkling details or
whimsical embroideries
are ultra-feminine.

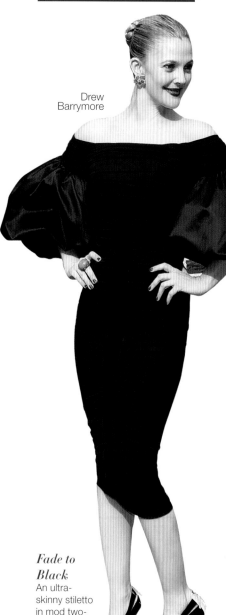

Drew
Barrymore

*Fade to
Black*
An ultra-
skinny stiletto
in mod two-
tone makes
a strikingly
strong point.

{3Os}

Now's the time to add some
dressed-up heels to your
collection of whimsical wares

• **Any way you want.** Addicted
to shoes? Far be it for us to
intervene. Every woman on
Earth is unique, and there are
shoes enough for each. The best
part is you don't have to buy
into just one style.

• **Bring a spare whenever you
can.** The Working Girl who
wears sneakers to work and
then switches into pumps is an
iconic image. But a chicer way
of making that commute more
comfortable is swapping those
Reeboks for ballet slippers.
They take up less space in your
bag, too.

• **What shoes go with your
jeans?** An ankle-length jean calls
for a flat or gladiator sandal,
while a longer leg needs a heel.

A glitzy stiletto can actually
turn your favorite pair of blues
into dressy party fare.

• **There's good cleavage and
bad.** A hint of a well-polished
toe is ultra-sexy. A satin
peep-toe will achieve a
suggestive look without being
trashy. But a sandal or mule
that shows too much of your
toes can make your foot look
ungainly and unfeminine.

• **Get in shape.** Some seasons
the runways herald rounded
toes; the next time around,
looks are pointed. Either way,
there's a stylish middle ground
for you—a little bit of both.
Just don't go in for super-sharp
looks, the sort that resemble
witches' boots.

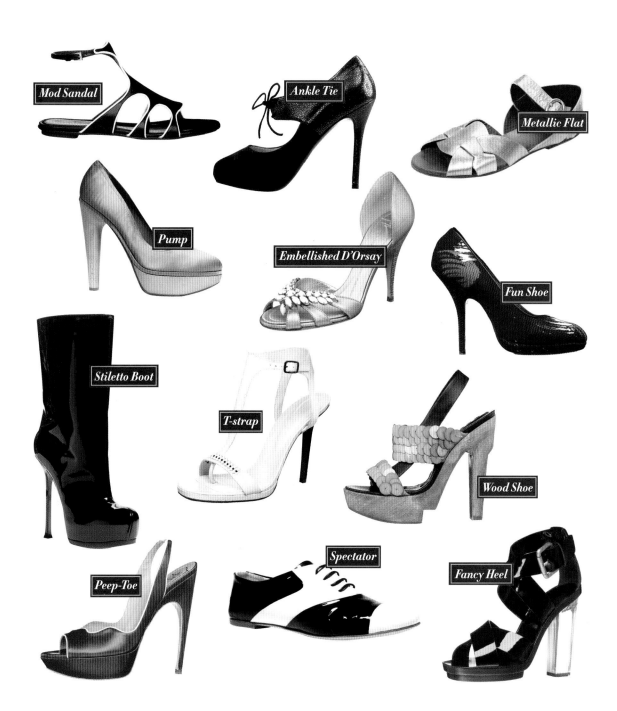

Mod Sandal

Ankle Tie

Metallic Flat

Pump

Embellished D'Orsay

Fun Shoe

Stiletto Boot

T-strap

Wood Shoe

Peep-Toe

Spectator

Fancy Heel

Skin Show A hint of toe, an exposed heel, a bare arch—scintillating.

Merry Mary-Jane The girl's shoe grows up and looks gorgeous.

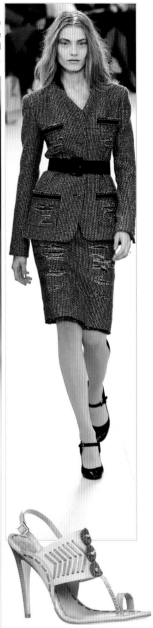

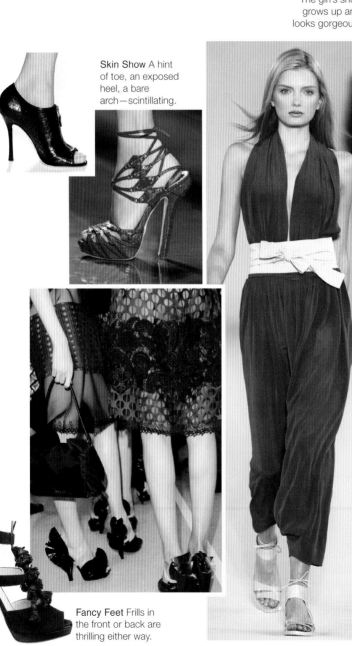

Fancy Feet Frills in the front or back are thrilling either way.

Sunny Sandals Whether flat or with a stiletto, they're great for days away.

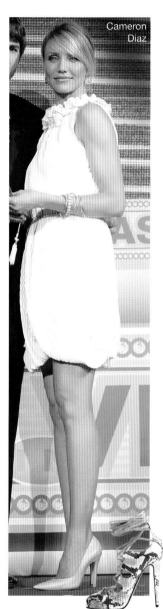

Cameron
Diaz

Jennifer
Connelly

Katie
Holmes

In the Tribe
Piling disparate motifs—floral
and ethnic, above and below—
is fashion-forward thinking.

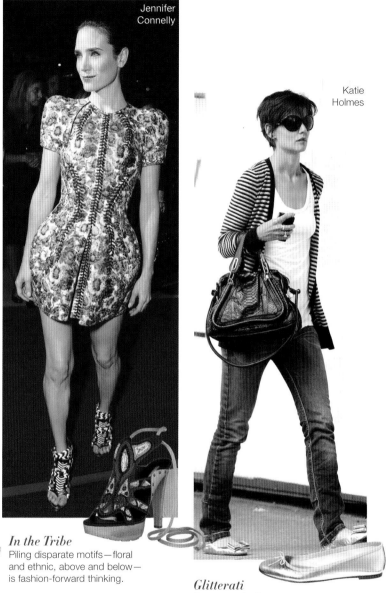

Barely There
A seemingly demure skin-tone
or snake shoe can make your
legs look long and sexily nude.

Glitterati
Even everyday jeans
and tees can use the
dazzle of a flashy shoe.

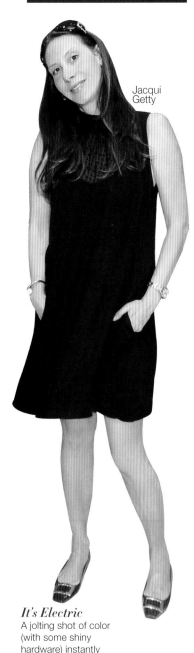

Jacqui
Getty

It's Electric
A jolting shot of color
(with some shiny
hardware) instantly
spruces up your basics.

{4Os}

Induldge in the transformative powers of footwear. In one week, you can be seven (or more) fabulous versions of yourself

• **Chunky heel or skinny heel?**
If you're a devoted shoe lover
who changes her looks with
the seasons, you are constantly
having to switch between a thick
heel and a slimmer one. The key
is buying the right kind of both
that will outlast fashion's whims.
A thicker heel is really only OK
if you have thinner calves and
ankles; otherwise, it will just
look clunky. On the other hand,
anyone can pull off a skinnier
shape that elongates the legs.

• **Maximize your shoe closet.**
In the summertime, a brown
leather sandal can be worn with
just about anything. It translates
in the winter, too, if you wear
tights. Opt for a chunkier look,
not one with thin straps.

• **Low can have impact, too.**
Dressed-up flats will give your
feet a rest but won't compromise
on the look you want to
achieve. A printed number will
make a pencil skirt pop or give
a flared skirt a vintage feel.

• **The last big fling.** Your biker
boots may have to veer toward
the more refined, but a good
buckle and perhaps fewer studs
(if any) are de rigeur now.

• **Explore the exotics, whether
real or fake, like croc and
snake.** They create instant visual
luxury and are—added bonus—
neutrals that go with pretty
much anything.

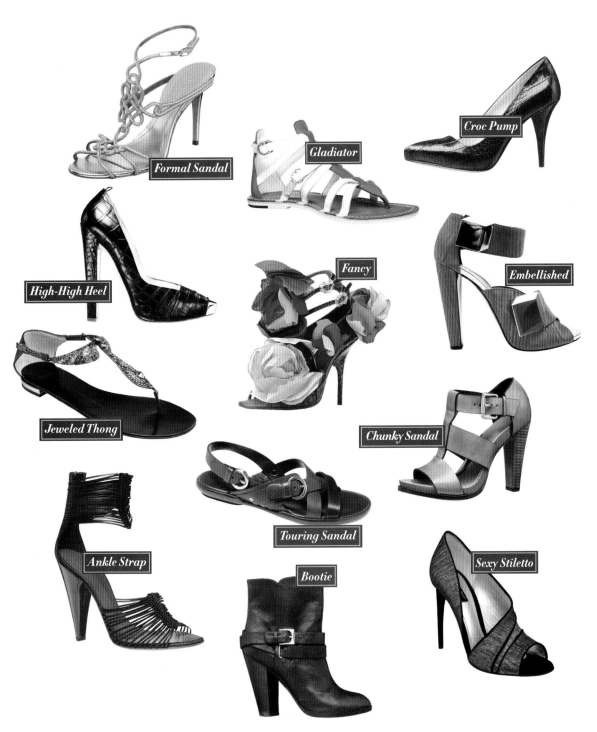

Formal Sandal

Gladiator

Croc Pump

High-High Heel

Fancy

Embellished

Jeweled Thong

Chunky Sandal

Ankle Strap

Touring Sandal

Bootie

Sexy Stiletto

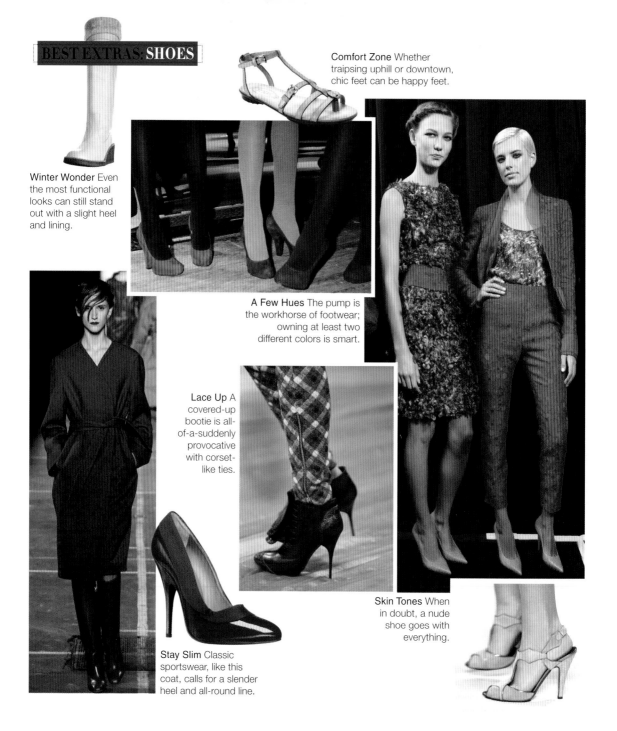

Comfort Zone Whether traipsing uphill or downtown, chic feet can be happy feet.

Winter Wonder Even the most functional looks can still stand out with a slight heel and lining.

A Few Hues The pump is the workhorse of footwear; owning at least two different colors is smart.

Lace Up A covered-up bootie is all-of-a-suddenly provocative with corset-like ties.

Stay Slim Classic sportswear, like this coat, calls for a slender heel and all-round line.

Skin Tones When in doubt, a nude shoe goes with everything.

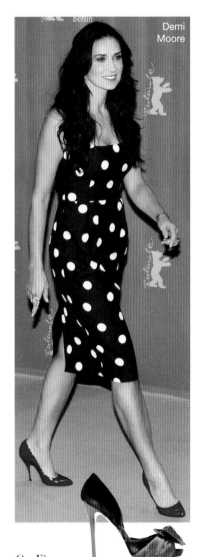

Demi Moore

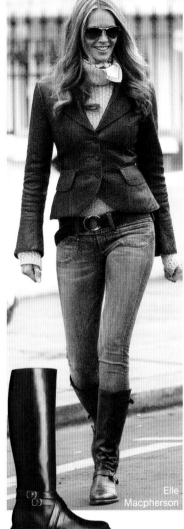

The Must-Own
Do you have a flat brown boot yet? It will quickly become your go-to.

Elle Macpherson

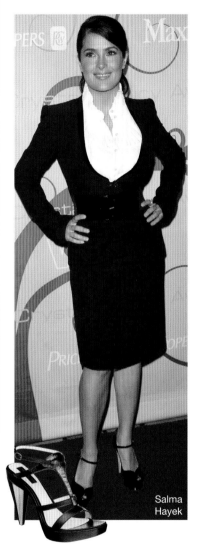

Salma Hayek

On Fire
It doesn't get sexier than a teetering skinny heel in cha-cha-cha red.

Great Heights
Slim platforms will give diminutive figures a much-needed boost.

{5os}

Put a pep in your step with traditional styles that have extra zing

• **Can you take it higher?** If you love to wear a high heel, indulge yourself. A thin stiletto can act like the punctuation mark to a stylish leg. The added height lengthens you and gives your calves a toned look.

• **The instant feel-good.** Whether it's to treat yourself or boost your mood, buying an awesome new piece of footwear is a fabulous thrill—and it will look great on any figure.

• **Patent will pump you up.** Like a perfectly lacquered toe, the shine of a closed-toe shoe in glossy leather can segue beautifully from the office to cocktails.

• **Add some jeweled boudoir-style beauties to your closet.** They slide on with the ease of slippers but are fancy enough for black-tie affairs.

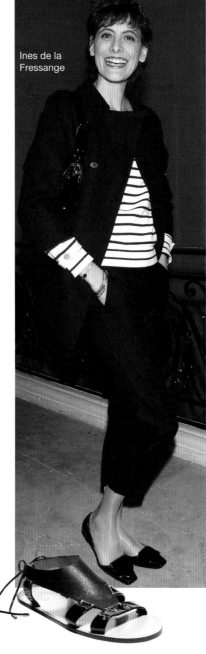

Ines de la Fressange

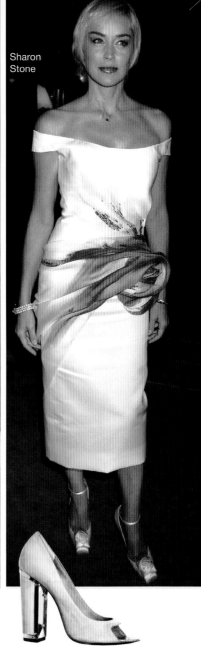

Sharon Stone

Pilgrim's Progress
Details like big buckles and laces aren't just for school girls. They make chic flats for grownups. And a little patent will dress it up.

In Neutral
A hushed tone will let your evening dress make the statement. Choose an ankle strap or thicker heel for added support.

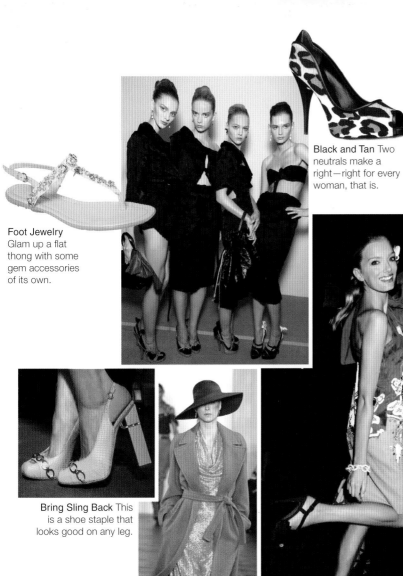

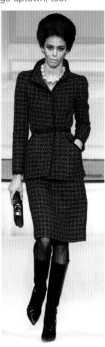

To the Point Black boots aren't just for Hell's Angels. They go uptown, too.

Black and Tan Two neutrals make a right—right for every woman, that is.

Foot Jewelry Glam up a flat thong with some gem accessories of its own.

Bring Sling Back This is a shoe staple that looks good on any leg.

Love the Ballet Getting around in comfort can be done in style, too.

Strap Happy Thin lines are a delicate and lovely way to stay secure.

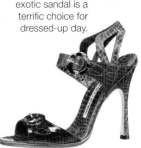

Croc Rocks An exotic sandal is a terrific choice for dressed-up day.

{60s}

Indulge in the creative possibilities of shoes: rich metallics, vivid hues, and sexy heels are like portable little works of art

• **Show some skin.** An ankle, the arch of a foot, a little bit of toe cleavage, there's more than one way to bare it.

• **Black is the new brown**—a black knee-high boot is the stylish workhorse of your wardrobe, able to pull together a skirt or dress outfit as easily as it does jeans.

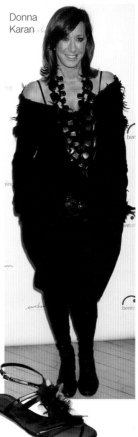

Donna Karan

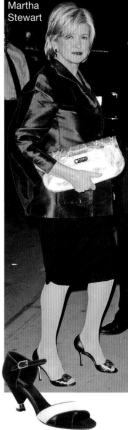

Martha Stewart

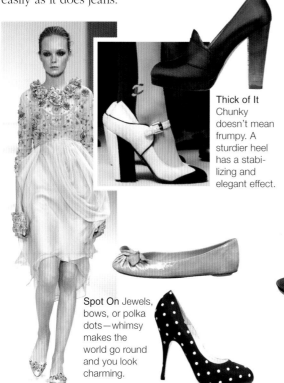

Thick of It Chunky doesn't mean frumpy. A sturdier heel has a stabilizing and elegant effect.

Spot On Jewels, bows, or polka dots—whimsy makes the world go round and you look charming.

Fleet Flat
To look effortless even when dressed up, don black knee-high leather boots or slip into a playful sandal.

Elegant Classic
The D'Orsay pump is fabled for revealing the sexy arch of a woman's foot. Add a strap for more security.

{70+}

Sky-high shoes aren't the only way to flatter your legs. Kitten heels and slim flats keep you sophisticated and au courant

White-Tie Event
Bows (not too floppy) and a cluster of baubles make great accents.

The Wee One
A tiny heel with a longer sandal toe or a skin-tone pump is lovely for day.

• **You can fake extra inches with a wedge or platform.** They look best as sandals that create a balanced counterpoint to a thick base.

• **If you must go high, go bold.** After all, everyone loves an amazing piece of footwear, and we all know we wear our shoes for other women's benefit.

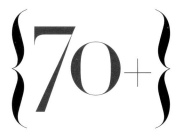
Shirley Bassey

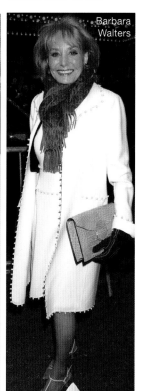
Barbara Walters

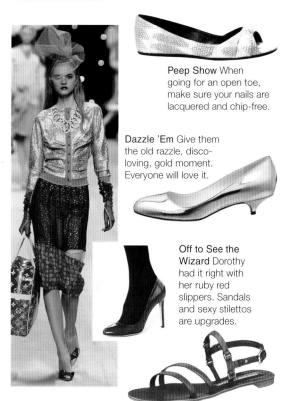

Peep Show When going for an open toe, make sure your nails are lacquered and chip-free.

Dazzle 'Em Give them the old razzle, disco-loving, gold moment. Everyone will love it.

Off to See the Wizard Dorothy had it right with her ruby red slippers. Sandals and sexy stilettos are upgrades.

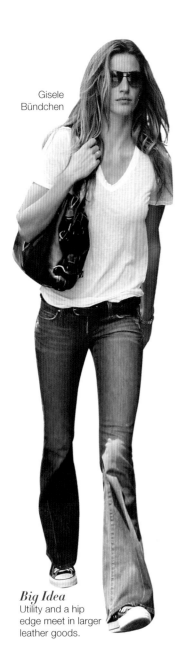

Gisele
Bündchen

Big Idea
Utility and a hip
edge meet in larger
leather goods.

{20s}
Bags

Think of a bag as an extension of your personality,
a calling card of stylish flair right at your fingertips

• **There are so many to choose from.** How to narrow it down? What you actually need are the following: an everyday tote in a neutral, a fun weekend clutch, and an elegant evening bag—plus don't forget your wallet.

• **If you're in the mood for kooky cool, now is the time to let loose a little.** Eye-popping colors, wacky appliqués, and off-kilter shapes can look charming.

• **Can I get that supersized?** Bags, like women, come in all shapes and sizes. You can tote around a card-holder-size number or envelope wallet, or you can lug a giant hobo style,

the sort that could feasibly carry a few pairs of shoes, a trendy pet, or a small child (not that we endorse the latter two).

• **Where do you stand on logos?** While every few years there's a no-go-logo movement, the pendulum eventually swings back to embrace them. So it's safe to buy something with your favorite label's mark on it, though it may have to rest in its dust bag every now and then.

• **Your new business cards deserve a safe place.** If you can splurge a little, a classy little case will save you having to reach into your pocket after a meeting.

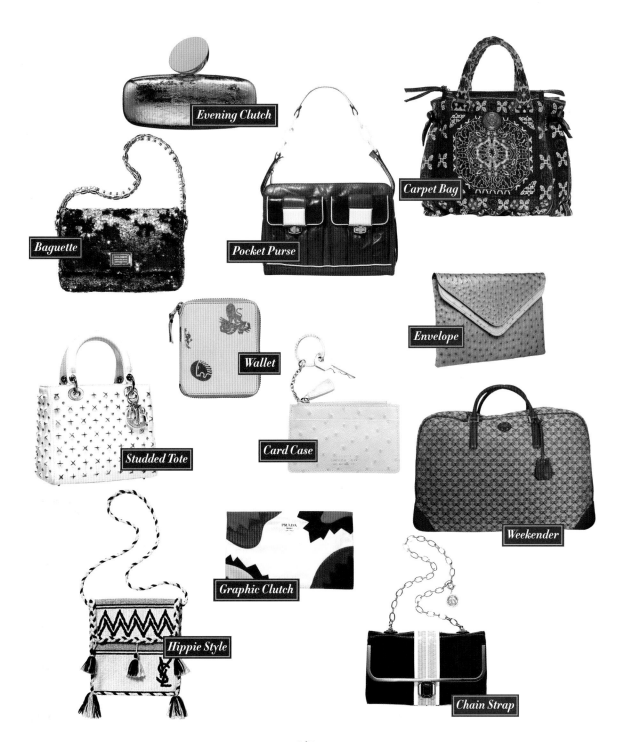

Evening Clutch

Carpet Bag

Baguette

Pocket Purse

Wallet

Envelope

Studded Tote

Card Case

Weekender

Graphic Clutch

Hippie Style

Chain Strap

Ladies Who Will
Lunch Practice polish
and refinement now
with trim shapes.

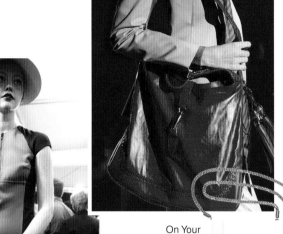

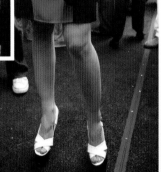

On Your
Shoulder
Lugging these
great shapes
around is
no problem.

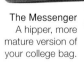

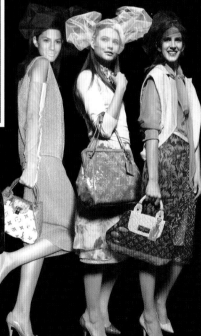

The Messenger
A hipper, more
mature version of
your college bag.

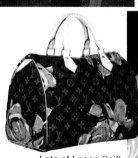

Lots of Logos Spiff
up the popular
brand names with
hot hues and humor.

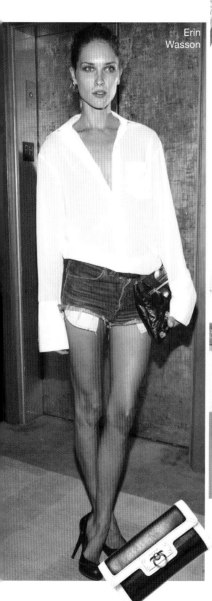

Erin
Wasson

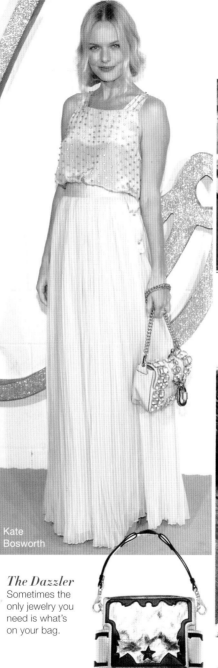

Kate
Bosworth

Rachel
Bilson

Metal Works
Tough hardware against a black
backdrop is surprisingly versatile
with both laidback and ladylike.

The Dazzler
Sometimes the
only jewelry you
need is what's
on your bag.

Red Alert
A pop of color will
elevate an otherwise
muted ensemble.

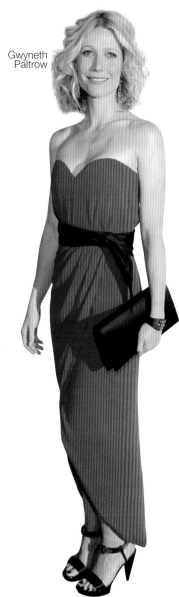

Gwyneth Paltrow

{30s}

Now is the time to toy around with different shapes, sizes, colors, and patterns

• **Old is new again.** The saying is never truer than when it comes to bags. Roomy doctors' holdalls, beaded baguettes, dazzling minaudières, and quilted looks (vintage or brand new) still look modern and fresh today.

• **Imagine a metallic bag as arm candy.** It comes in silver or gold leather wrapping, and its great taste will last as long as you want it to.

• **Rethink the term "strap-hanger."** It takes on a whole new meaning when you consider how diverse the traditional day look has become. Chains, ropes, knots, even the odd arc of resin can hook on your shoulder for easy wear.

• **First class all the way.** Even if you're in coach—who can travel up front anyway, these days?—you can still travel with style. A bigger, strappy bag can safely store a sweater, magazines, and your computer. Also look out for pockets—they will keep your tickets, keys, and cell from becoming a messy pile at the bottom.

• **Ditch the backpack.** They're for high schoolers and college travelers.

• **Don't ignore the basics.** You don't always have time to switch bags when you change outfits, so for those occasions, make sure you have something versatile, like a monochrome or skin.

Grab Bag
A simple black clutch is all you need to get you through the night.

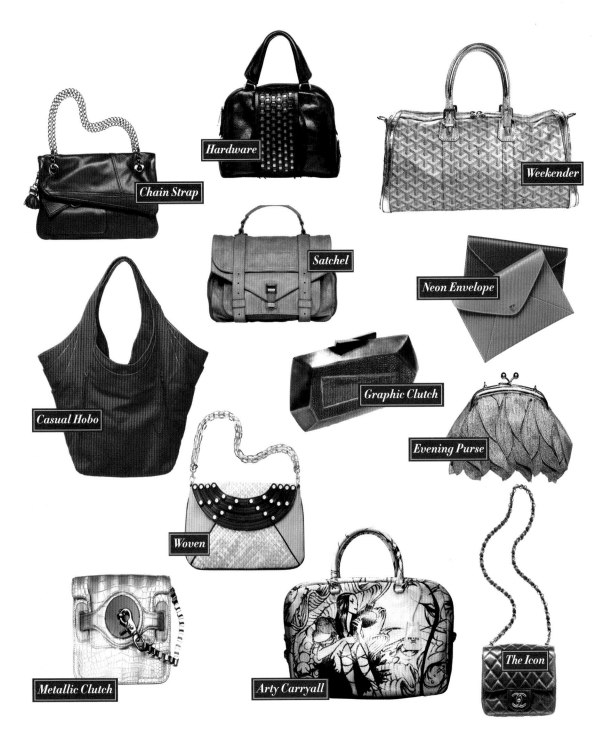

Chain Strap

Hardware

Weekender

Satchel

Neon Envelope

Casual Hobo

Graphic Clutch

Evening Purse

Woven

Metallic Clutch

Arty Carryall

The Icon

Stripes and Stuff Colors and patterns are a sure-fire way to get noticed.

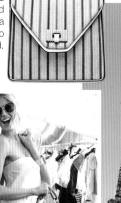

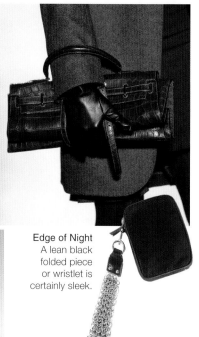

Edge of Night A lean black folded piece or wristlet is certainly sleek.

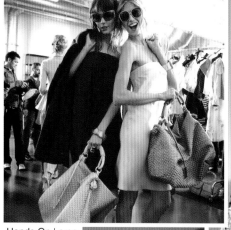

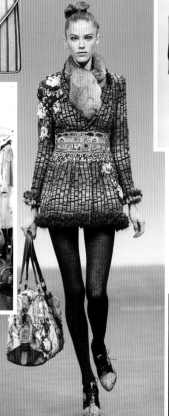

Hands On Large and roomy or small and sporty, it's chic to swing these beauties around town.

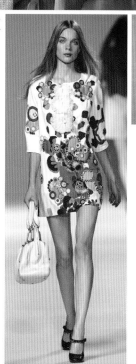

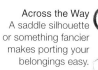

Across the Way A saddle silhouette or something fancier makes porting your belongings easy.

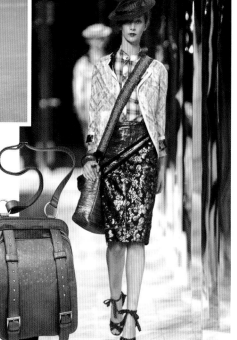

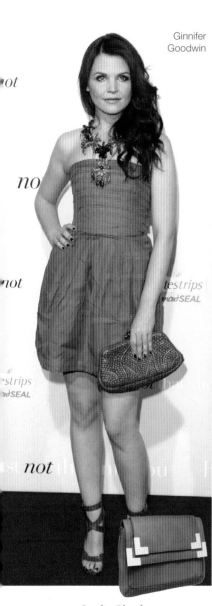

Ginnifer Goodwin

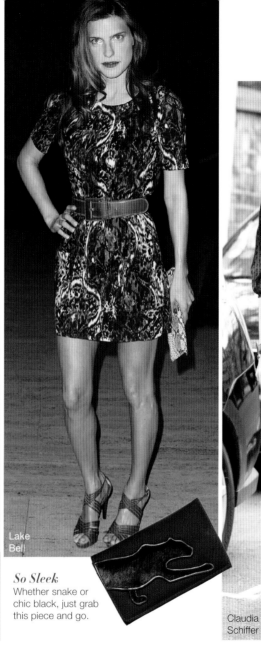

Lake Bell

So Sleek
Whether snake or chic black, just grab this piece and go.

In the Shade
Tonal gradations from jewelry to dress to bag to shoe are subtle and sophisticated.

Claudia Schiffer

Pleat Fleet
There are all kinds of details. Folds— or a pop of neon—turn a brown leather tote into something crafty.

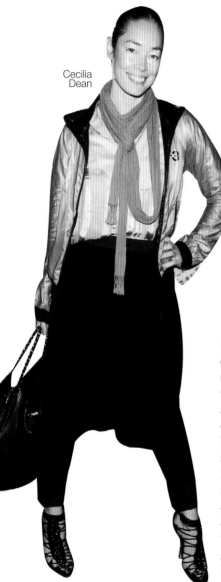

Cecilia Dean

Hot Hobo
Urban hippies love the mixed-up motif of a voluminous, slouchy sac.

{40s}

Your dust bags are safeguarding an eclectic mélange of old, new, classic, and colorful

• **If you're packing for a short getaway, the last thing you need is a clunky suitcase.** A weekender is the stylish solution. The straps are easy on your shoulder, and the body big enough for a few ensembles and shoes, plus a good book. If you're gone for a week or more, you definitely need a sturdy set of luggage. Opt for something other than black, though. There are plenty of gorgeous pieces that are beautiful, easy to spot on the endlessly looping bag carousel, and practical (with wheels).

• **The bag you've all been waiting for.** Admit it: even if you don't play into labels, there are those iconic shapes and silhouettes that hover in your sartorial psyche. They're generally expensive (but worth it since most appreciate well and last for decades). You're old enough to carry them with poise, and you may have a wee bit of cash saved up for investments (remember cost per wear). So go ahead and treat yourself to that lovely, enduring present.

• **Stud-ly do right.** It's great to go in for some substantial hardware, like smaller spikes, ornate filigree, or other graphic metal details.

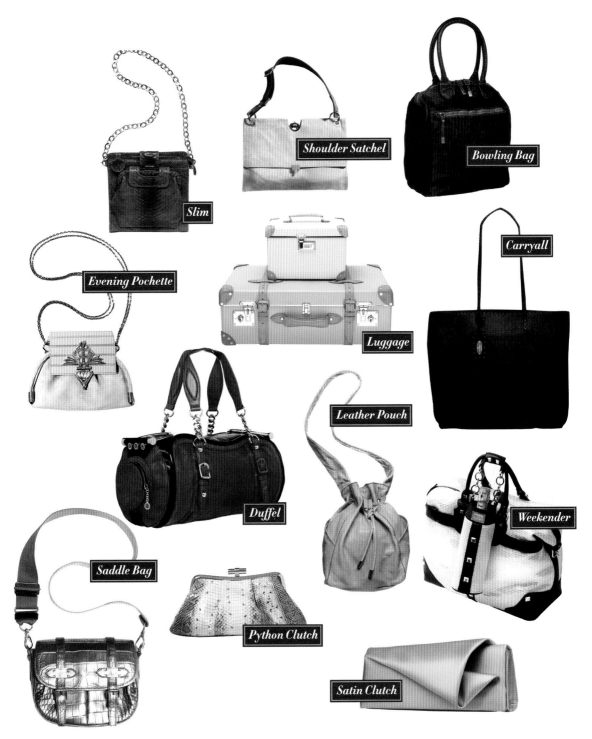

Slim

Shoulder Satchel

Bowling Bag

Evening Pochette

Luggage

Carryall

Duffel

Leather Pouch

Weekender

Saddle Bag

Python Clutch

Satin Clutch

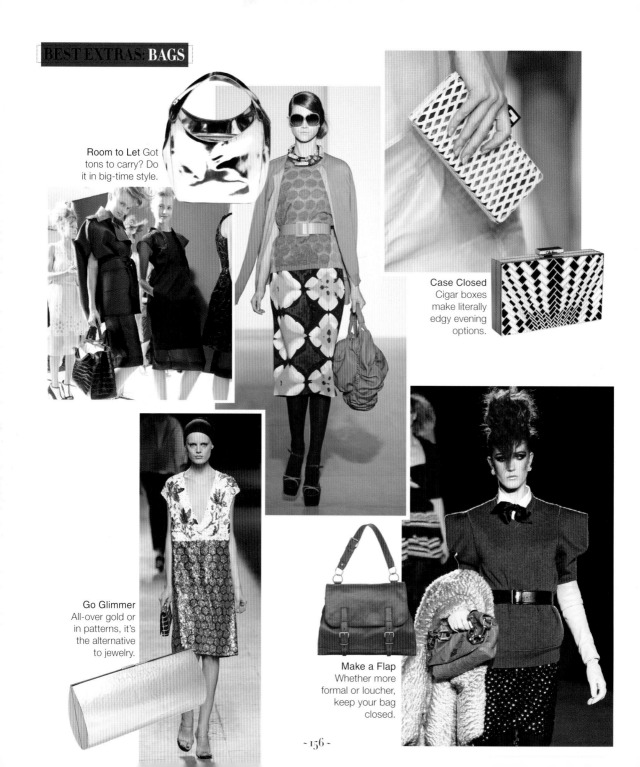

Room to Let Got tons to carry? Do it in big-time style.

Case Closed Cigar boxes make literally edgy evening options.

Go Glimmer All-over gold or in patterns, it's the alternative to jewelry.

Make a Flap Whether more formal or loucher, keep your bag closed.

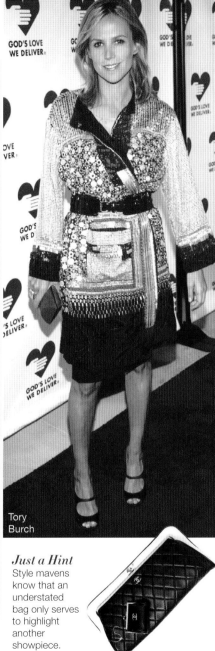

Carla Bruni-Sarkozy

Tory Burch

Sandra Bullock

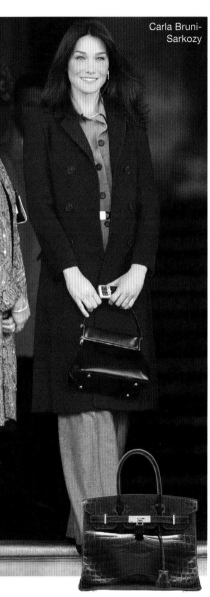

The Icons
They don't call them that for nothing—always quietly phenomenal.

Just a Hint
Style mavens know that an understated bag only serves to highlight another showpiece.

On the Go
In a rush, a clutch carries everything you need for a night on the town.

{50s}

Extreme details have given way to more refined and luxe options

• **Don't leave your sense of humor at home.** A frill, a feather, a clutch full of flou: a vibrant, quirky item can be a great conversation starter. And best of all, it still holds your phone, wallet, and favorite lipstick.

• **Classically quirky may as well be its own category.** Blending a traditional bag with cool detailing is one way of having your cake and eating it, too. Think about unusual shades to brighten things up, or do a neutral leather or croc in an unexpected silhouette. Either way, you'll stand out.

• **It's like jewelry—but for your bag.** A little hardware—semi-precious stones, metal grommets, mesh chains, or heavy embroidery—will win you second glances. If your tote speaks volumes, though, tone down the other accessories.

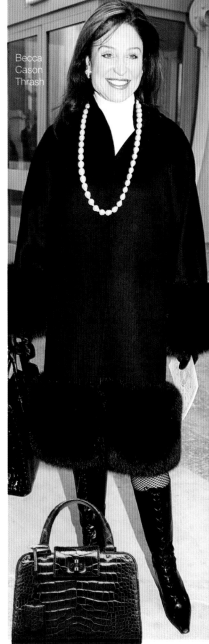

Becca
Cason
Thrash

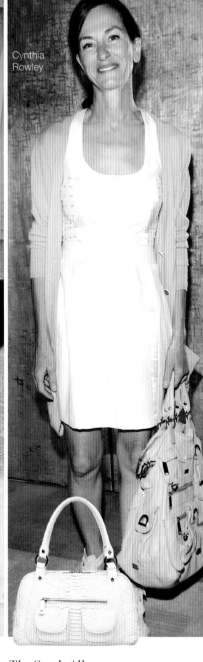

Cynthia
Rowley

Classical Arts
A string of pearls, a luxe trim, and the most graceful of bags—it's an arresting combination.

The Catch-All
The modern woman carries a lot. But a louche leather piece with tons of pockets keeps her looking fine no matter what.

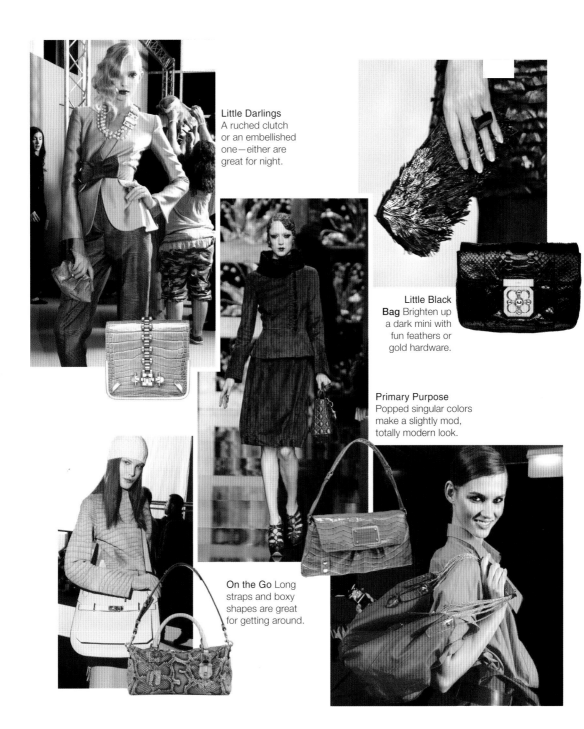

Little Darlings
A ruched clutch
or an embellished
one—either are
great for night.

**Little Black
Bag** Brighten up
a dark mini with
fun feathers or
gold hardware.

Primary Purpose
Popped singular colors
make a slightly mod,
totally modern look.

On the Go Long
straps and boxy
shapes are great
for getting around.

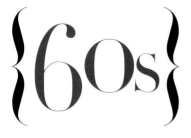

{60s}

Your days are split between practicality and revelry; you're closet should be, too—from a killer day tote to a dazzling evening clutch

• **Is your personality fierce and fearless or sweet and polished?** A little bit of both, right? Thankfully, bags allow you to switch gears with minimal fuss.

• **Fade to background.** Sometimes your tote, pouch, or envelope needs to be all but invisible. Black makes a great option, but so does an embossed croc or burnished metallic.

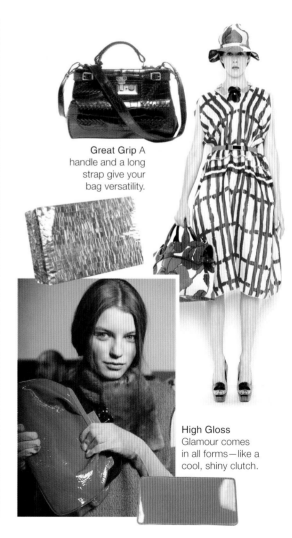

Great Grip A handle and a long strap give your bag versatility.

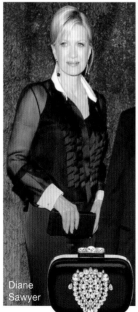

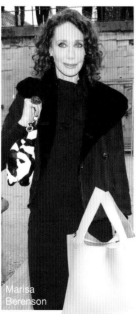

Diane Sawyer

Marisa Berenson

High Gloss Glamour comes in all forms—like a cool, shiny clutch.

Nights in Black Satin
A clutch that flows seamlessly with your overall ensemble is a mark of true glamour.

Ebony and Ivory
Sometimes all you need is a little visual contrast to keep things lively.

{70+}

Sit back and enjoy a bevy of beautiful, old, sophisticated wonders that you've collected and smartly stored

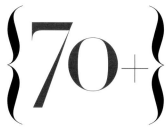

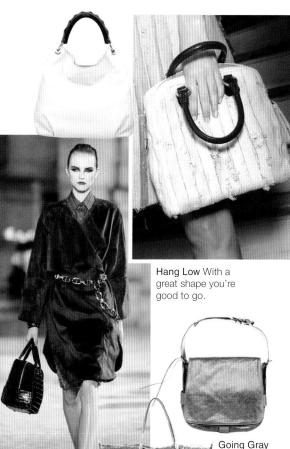

Hang Low With a great shape you're good to go.

Going Gray A metallic or muted silver is the height of polished chic.

• **Start your day with a jingle and a jangle.** Day looks can be just as detailed as event pieces. The difference is the size—larger is obviously a must.

• **Zip it, button it, or lock it.** Closures can be like miniature works of art. A good one not only keeps your belongings safe but also serves as a creative focal point.

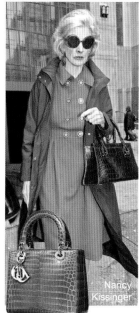

Nancy Kissinger

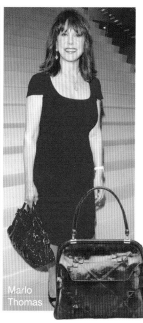

Marlo Thomas

Classic Cool
Square shapes give form to your overall look and are best for day.

Hot Topic
A dash of red or any other bright jewel tone will spark in all the right ways.

Scarves

No longer just for cold weather, this versatile accessory is now stepping out in all seasons

• **Looped, knotted, tied, doubled-up or left hanging?** Worn different ways, the same scarf can be reincarnated over and over. One day it looks artfully messy; the next it is a polished finishing touch. A great-value buy.

• **The louchest of layers.** For street-chic lovers they're part of the daily uniform of tee, sweater, jacket, jeans, scarf. This is the archetypal effortless ensemble.

• **Something that cradles your face** should be as soft and gentle as the finest lotion. Materials like silk, cashmere, and cottons washed in milk (yes, milk) feel like pure heaven.

• **Not just for necks.** Look for fresh ways to style them: wrapped around your wrist or tied on your bag.

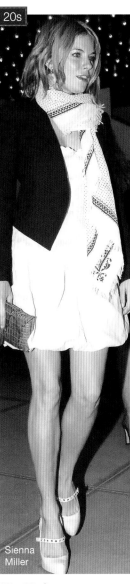

20s

Sienna Miller

Hot Nights
Even dressed-up dolls need to stay warm. A nonchalantly thrown-on swath is the height of stylish ease.

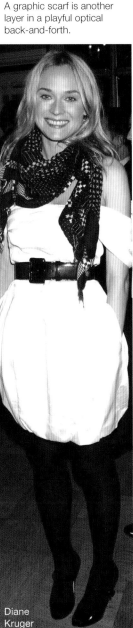

In Reverse
Black-white-black-white. A graphic scarf is another layer in a playful optical back-and-forth.

Diane Kruger

30s

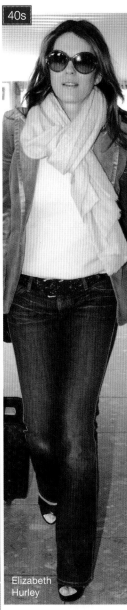

40s

Elizabeth Hurley

Nude Number
A pale tone in cashmere is an everyday luxury. It's beautiful but not so loud it overpowers.

Deep Purple
A rich jewel tone plays well against a simpler, neutral ensemble—and keeps you toasty.

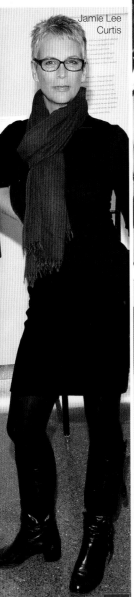

Jamie Lee Curtis

60s

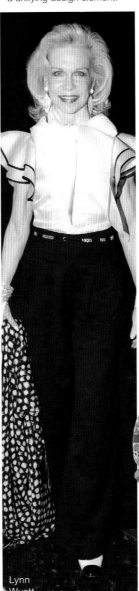

Diane von Furstenberg

Bunched Up
Louche knows no age limit. A casual wrap-and-tie is a multi-dimensional bonus. And now, the fabric is luxe.

Class Mates
A larger pashmina-like style will not only be a chic cover-up, but it can also be a unifying design element.

Lynn Wyatt

Editors' Picks

Hippie Heaven
Popping up your colors is always a smart idea.

Ooh La La
Traditional French motifs will never ever look dated and add a polished, bright accent to a muted outfit.

Cotton Comfort
Don't you want to pillow your face in the softest materials?

Pattern Party
A lively palette is a great substitute for days when you don't wear jewelry.

Ethereal Embroidery
Far-off embellishments will make you look wonderfully worldly.

50s

70+

Belts

All women want a defined waist, so whatever your age, make a cincher an integral part of your look

• **Both functional and fabulously fashionable.** With so many variations, this piece serves as much as a statement of your personal style—there's life beyond the simple black leather belt—as a way to flatter your figure.

• **The shape shifter.** Belts, thin or thick, are the simplest and quickest way to define your body and reproportion you. They give sack dresses structure and draw attention to the smallest part of your body—a wonderful ability, if you ask us.

• **What's best for me?** If you have a short torso, a thinner belt will pull you in while simultaneously masking your lack of length. A thicker belt, on the other hand, will help those blessed with long midriffs balance out their upper and lower halves.

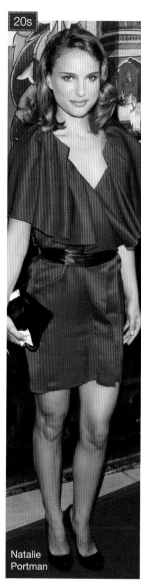

20s

Natalie Portman

A Ribbon Will Do
When you maximize volume above or below, you need a sliver of something—like a satin sash—to rein it in.

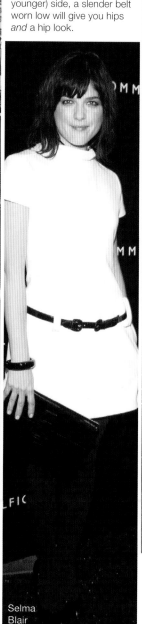

Miss Mod
If you're on the slimmer (and younger) side, a slender belt worn low will give you hips *and* a hip look.

Selma Blair

30s

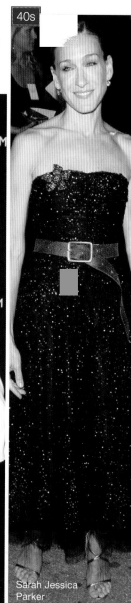

40s

Sarah Jessica Parker

The Odd Couple
Age breeds confidence and brilliant fashion choices—a rugged belt with an evening look.

A Kinder Corset
Wide belts are contouring. They have a girdling effect that keeps your waist looking trim and long.

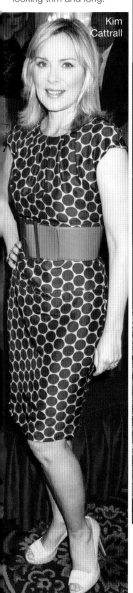

Kim Cattrall

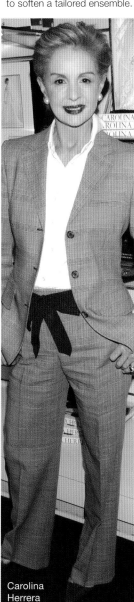

Diane Keaton

Add a Coat
Too-pretty, too-trendy belts look age-awkward. But a substantial leather piece is spot on.

Center Piece
A larger, floppier bow—as opposed to a small, sweet one—is an unexpected way to soften a tailored ensemble.

Carolina Herrera

Editors' Picks

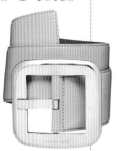

Brighten Up A vibrantly hued cincher can jazz up just about anything.

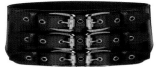

Hard Edge A tough, multi-buckle look is sexiest when paired with something simple or ladylike.

Triple Threat A coiled belt has that same effortless, piled-on appeal as a wrapped necklace or bracelet.

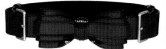

Buckles Count Closures, like a jaunty bowtie or a jeweled marvel, can have design flair.

On Safari Canvas, jute, or rope styles have great texture and are neutrals that go with everything.

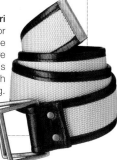

{20s} Jewelry

Your jewelry picks are bold, colorful, and charmingly off-kilter

• **Good things come in multiples.** Piling on the glittering chains, rings, and bracelets creates texture and an air of effortless styling.

• **That's odd(ly beautiful).** Real or costume, get resourceful and creative with your jewelry. Think about using gold coins as earrings, vintage buttons as charms, and so on.

Flirty Flowers Think of it as a corsage for your neck.

Mixed Motif A pastiche of stones will complement various looks.

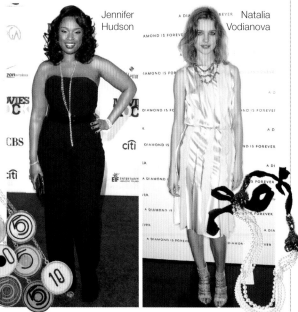

Jennifer Hudson

Natalia Vodianova

Hard Rock Tons of chains, big beads, and chunky rings are totally tough.

Chain Gang
Lariats aren't just for cowgirls. They're ultra-hip—or add charms for quirkiness.

First Pearls
Artfully splayed gray beauties or multiple strings are a fresh take on the classic.

{30s}

Like a fashion magpie, collect gems, jewels, and baubles on your travels; they'll serve as stylish reminders of good times and adventures

Wrist Watch A gorgeous timepiece or jeweled bracelet is grown-up and dressed-up.

• **Look like a maharani.** Indian-inspired costume jewelry makes you look rich even if the stones are made from glass. And the colors and intricate craftsmanship are attention-getters.

• **Not everything should be in-your-face fabulous.** Gentler pieces, like ribbon-anchored necklaces or refined watches, are just as important.

All that Glitters A strong ring design is a wonderful piece to own for years.

Don Doodads Bold and big or delightful and delicate, drop earrings are a must.

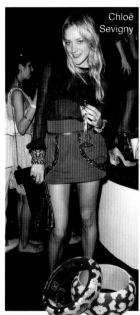

Chloë Sevigny

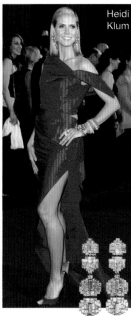

Heidi Klum

Smart Buys Wood or resin cuffs are a sensational but more budget-friendly look.

Beautiful Bunch Irreverently piling on silver jewelry is a cool way to defuss evening.

{ 40s }

Things are getting dramatic. Your collection is a brilliant brew of wild, elegant, and all-round dazzling pieces

• **Being chunky is actually a good thing.** Large, demonstrative looks can often anchor your entire ensemble, like a substantial, sculpted gold cuff played against a stark black dress.

• **Something old, something new.** Adding vintage-like gems and edgier fare to your jewelry box is a modern way to dress.

Moon Rock
Oversized rings are a trend that's here to stay.

Giant Gems
Big in size and in style, they scream luxury (even if they're faux).

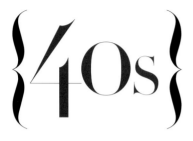

Julianne Moore

Kristen Scott Thomas

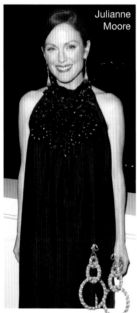

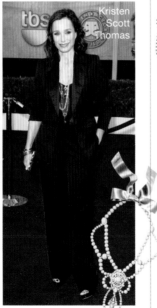

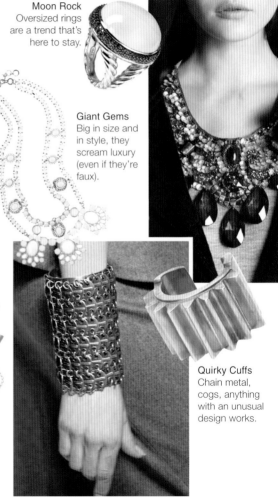

Quirky Cuffs
Chain metal, cogs, anything with an unusual design works.

Drop It
Tear-drop earrings will earn you raves and draw attention to your face.

Gorgeous Gaggle
Layers and layers of thin gold chains or a beaded necklace work best against black.

{5OS}

You own larger-than-life jewels in artistic shapes and big-time stones. Even if they're not real, their size is

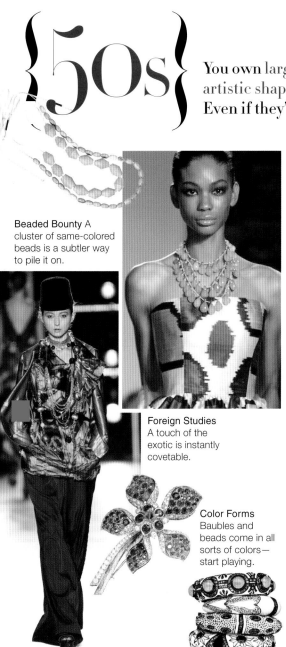

Beaded Bounty A cluster of same-colored beads is a subtler way to pile it on.

Foreign Studies A touch of the exotic is instantly covetable.

Color Forms Baubles and beads come in all sorts of colors—start playing.

• **Mother Nature does it best.** Don't underestimate the beauty of floral or faunal motifs re-created with a glittering stone or lacquer. They're simply lovely.

• **Wood works wonderfully, too.** The arts and crafts movement lives on in exciting baubles with artisanal finishes.

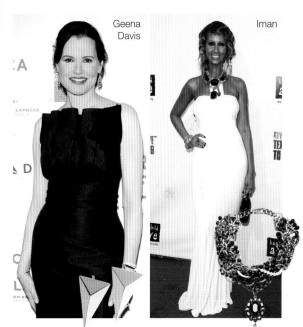

Geena Davis

Iman

Just a Drop
Keep them all dangling with a longer earring—whether teardrop or spiked.

Daring Dazzlers
If you've got an elegant neck and the moxie to pull it off, bulky can be brilliant.

{6Os}

Class and elegance should be your focus. Everything you own, even your artier and edgier goods, ooze sophistication

• **Time flies no matter what you're doing, so why not look amazing on the journey?** Watches can act like functional, bedazzled bracelets.

• **This one's from Kenya; this one's from Brazil.** Let your accessories be like the United Nations of style. Global effects are vastly interesting—and open up a world of styling possibilities.

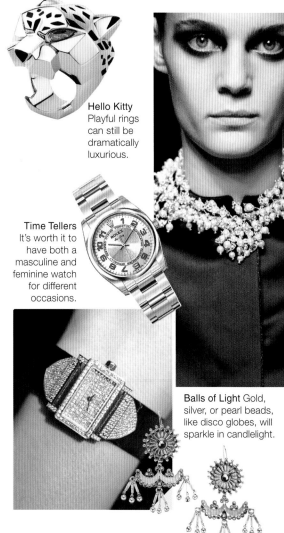

Hello Kitty
Playful rings can still be dramatically luxurious.

Time Tellers
It's worth it to have both a masculine and feminine watch for different occasions.

Balls of Light Gold, silver, or pearl beads, like disco globes, will sparkle in candlelight.

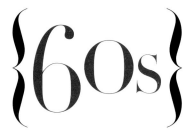

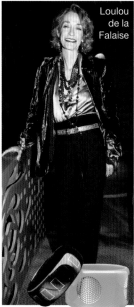

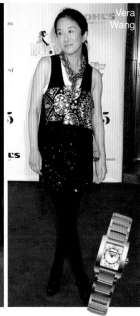

Loulou de la Falaise

Vera Wang

Palette Play
Your accessories should pick up on subtle colors within your outfit.

Silver and Gold
Throw out the old notion of never mixing metals. These two hues make a smashing duet.

{70+}

You wear the kind of enduring rings, earrings, cuffs, and chains that people find aspirational and inspirational

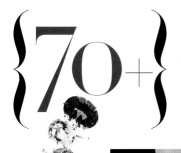

Circular Sensations
Softly rounded stones and jewelry are pleasing to the eye.

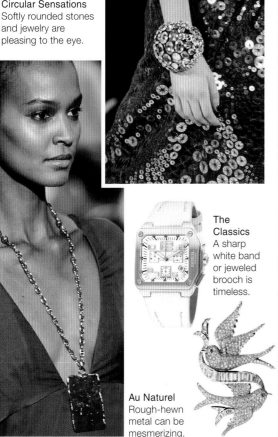

The Classics
A sharp white band or jeweled brooch is timeless.

Au Naturel
Rough-hewn metal can be mesmerizing.

• **As nature intended.** Precious and semi-precious stones are often most breathtaking when simply polished and set with no extras. Their color and clarity speak for themselves.

• **Go bold or go home.** Younger women can't always pull off bigger looks, like heaped-up necklaces or large brooches. You can and should.

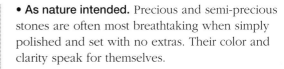

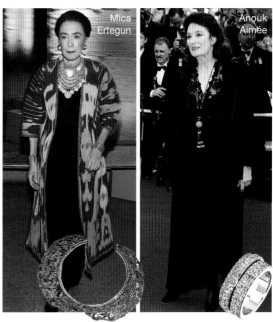

Mica Ertegun

Anouk Aimée

Treasure Chest
Like an Egyptian queen, extravagant gold necklaces are rightly regal.

Pretty and Polished
An elongated pendant lengthens your overall line, while a stacked ring will glisten.

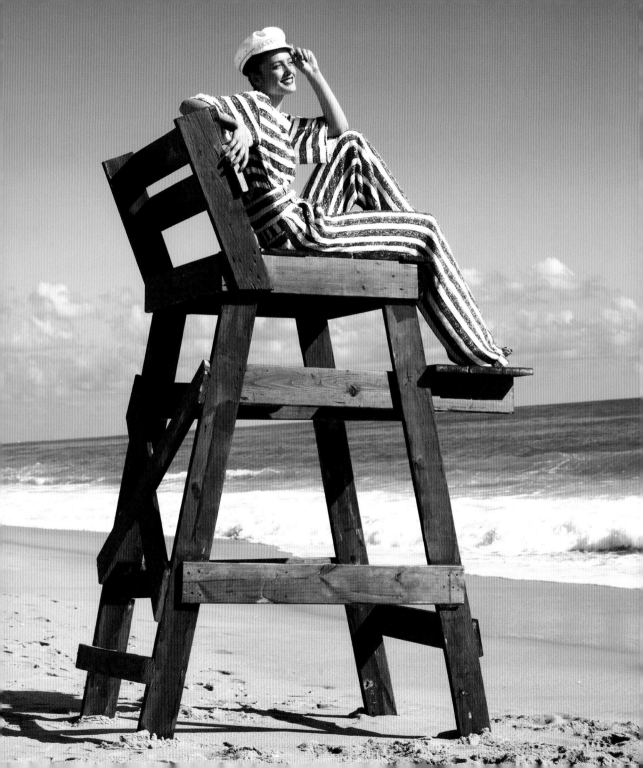

CHAPTER TEN

Beach Guide

Packing for a sunny holiday is delicate business. There are issues of space (in your suitcase) and shape (as in wearing a swimsuit in public). But confidence will be your greatest asset when heading off for warmer climes. Throw in some terrific sandals, fun sunglasses, and charming cover-ups

{ "Be smart about what you pack. Don't lug around ten extra suitcases because you couldn't make up your mind." —CHLOË SEVIGNY }

{20s}

Cool colors and silhouettes will help you stand out from the spring-breakers

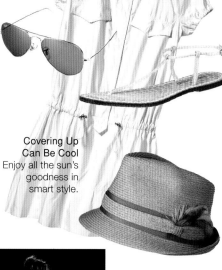

The Day Tote Pack everything you need in a chic carryall that's cheerful and sturdy.

Covering Up Can Be Cool Enjoy all the sun's goodness in smart style.

Bloomer Town A charming cover-up keeps you protected and pretty.

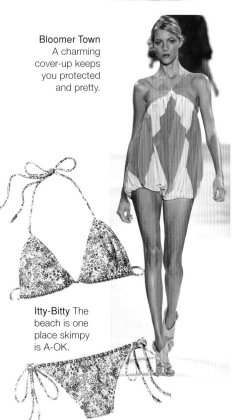

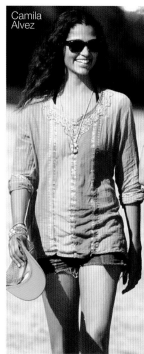

Camila Alvez

Cut Off Shredded jean shorts (you made them yourself) and a kurta are sandy-day musts.

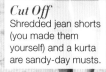

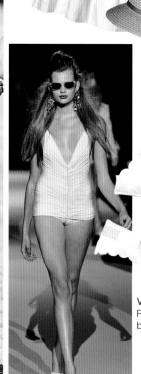

Vintage Mavens Retro looks can be sexy or sweet.

Itty-Bitty The beach is one place skimpy is A-OK.

{30s}

Sun-kissed sexiness is key with skimpy bikinis, glam extras, and fun cover-ups

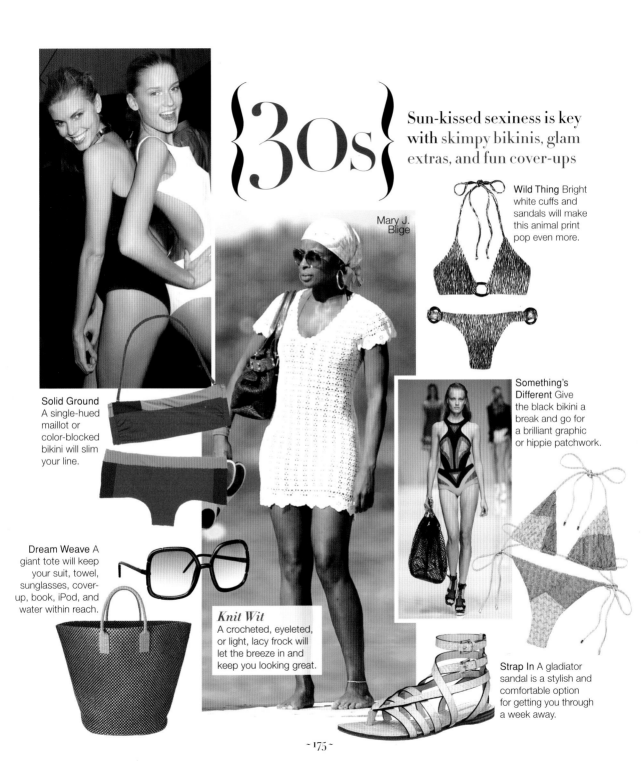

Wild Thing Bright white cuffs and sandals will make this animal print pop even more.

Mary J. Blige

Solid Ground A single-hued maillot or color-blocked bikini will slim your line.

Something's Different Give the black bikini a break and go for a brilliant graphic or hippie patchwork.

Dream Weave A giant tote will keep your suit, towel, sunglasses, cover-up, book, iPod, and water within reach.

Knit Wit
A crocheted, eyeleted, or light, lacy frock will let the breeze in and keep you looking great.

Strap In A gladiator sandal is a stylish and comfortable option for getting you through a week away.

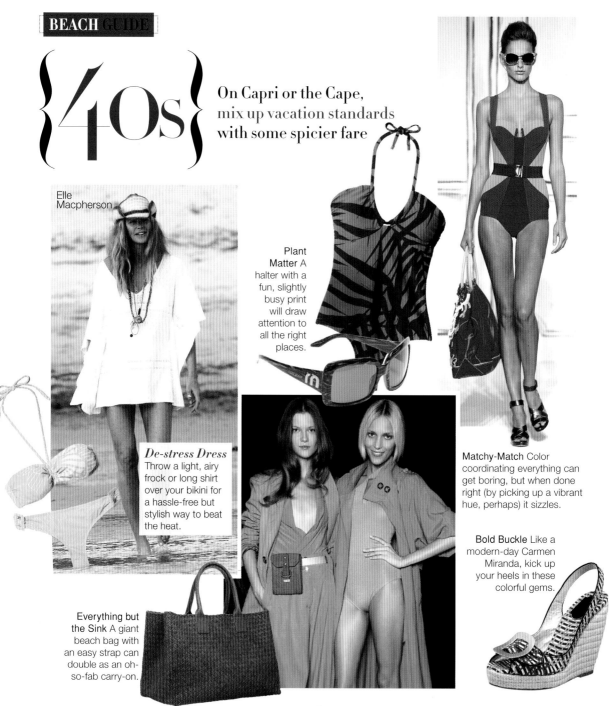

{40s}

On Capri or the Cape, mix up vacation standards with some spicier fare

Elle Macpherson

Plant Matter A halter with a fun, slightly busy print will draw attention to all the right places.

De-stress Dress Throw a light, airy frock or long shirt over your bikini for a hassle-free but stylish way to beat the heat.

Matchy-Match Color coordinating everything can get boring, but when done right (by picking up a vibrant hue, perhaps) it sizzles.

Bold Buckle Like a modern-day Carmen Miranda, kick up your heels in these colorful gems.

Everything but the Sink A giant beach bag with an easy strap can double as an oh-so-fab carry-on.

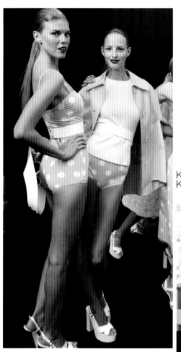

{50s}

If you've got it, flaunt it. But even then, keep thinking "age-appropriate"

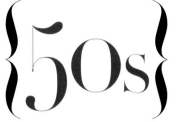

Kelly Klein

Suit Up If you're on the shyer side but still want to sizzle, try a boy-cut bikini.

Three Cheers Suits and cover-ups with a 1950s feel are a refreshing change of pace.

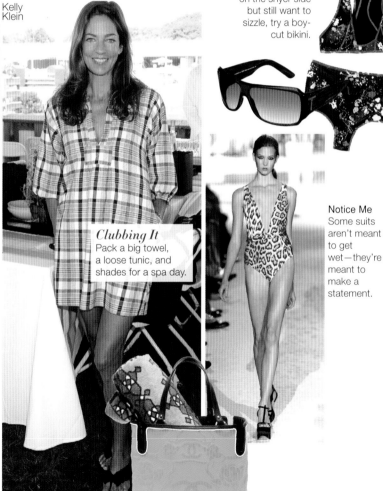

Clubbing It
Pack a big towel, a loose tunic, and shades for a spa day.

Notice Me Some suits aren't meant to get wet—they're meant to make a statement.

Earthy Girls Pairing Mother Nature's palette with a metallic is hot.

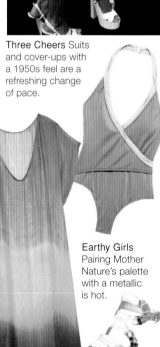

{60s}

If you're body conscious, there are plenty of styles that accentuate and camouflage

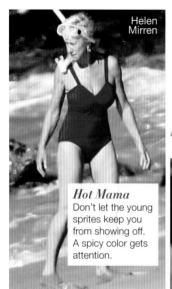

Helen Mirren

Top This A wide brim and a pastel print will charm.

Hot Mama
Don't let the young sprites keep you from showing off. A spicy color gets attention.

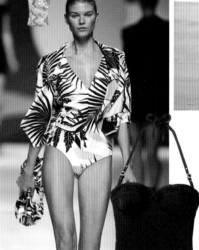

Like Trompe l'Oeil Smart color-blocking can fool others' eyes into seeing what you want them to see.

Knot's Landing A detailed metallic bag will look just as great at home, lowering its cost per wear.

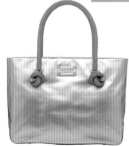

Best Mates A dark-light motif is easy for anyone to work.

All Aboard A boat shoe can be glam

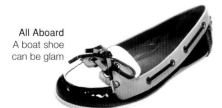

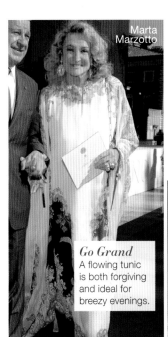
Marta Marzotto

{70+}

Soak up the rays the smart way—slightly covered up and sophisticated

Go Grand
A flowing tunic is both forgiving and ideal for breezy evenings.

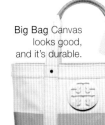

Jewel Joy
Even if you're stateside, little exotic touches are exciting.

Cinch In As always, a belt is the quickest way to give something— even a beach jacket—shape.

Greater Goods
The right shapes, colors and sizes will bring out your best.

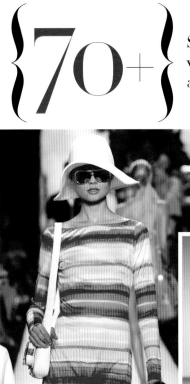

Shoulder Smolder A halter covers and reveals perfectly.

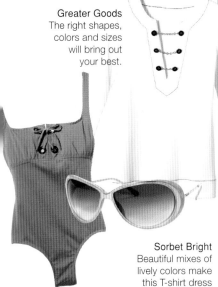

Sorbet Bright
Beautiful mixes of lively colors make this T-shirt dress beach-appropriate.

Big Bag Canvas looks good, and it's durable.

The Elements of Style

With the dizzying amount of new fashion that hits runways and stores every season (and pretty much in all the months in between), how do you keep track of what's necessary and what's not? We've thought long and hard about everything you have to juggle—work, social life, finances—while still staying true to your personality and figure. Yet we also know just how great it feels to indulge every once in a while in something that's just, well, pretty. So we've made a lot of suggestions on the previous pages in the hope that you will find plenty of options to suit you. But, just as a recap, we're going back to basics, with an easy-to-digest laundry list of what you should always have in your wardrobe no matter your age. From here, it's up to you.

3 Cardigans
*(1 neutral cashmere
1 colorful cashmere, 1 cotton)*

1 Suit
(skirt or pant)

3 Blouses
*(1 white button-down, 2 ladylike
or printed)*

1 Blazer
(navy or black)

4 T-Shirts
(1 white, 1 gray, 1 colored, 1 striped long-sleeve)

2 Pairs of Pants
(1 denim, 1 long trouser)

2 Coats
*(1 dressy cashmere,
1 day look)*

3 Skirts
*(1 black pencil, 1 embellished
pencil, 1 printed)*

2 Jackets
(1 leather, 1 cotton topper)

3 Dresses
(1 day, 1 evening, 1 LBD)

3 Bags
*(1 evening, 1 day carryall,
1 weekender)*

4 Pairs of Shoes
(1 sandal, 1 day pump, 1 brown boot, 1 evening)

Born to be Chic

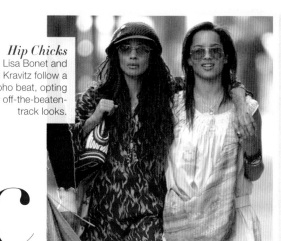

Hip Chicks
Lisa Bonet and
Zoë Kravitz follow a
boho beat, opting
for off-the-beaten-
track looks.

Like mother, like daughter. These stylish teams prove fashion savvy has nothing to do with age

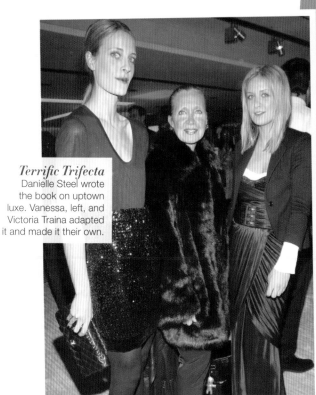

Terrific Trifecta
Danielle Steel wrote
the book on uptown
luxe. Vanessa, left, and
Victoria Traina adapted
it and made it their own.

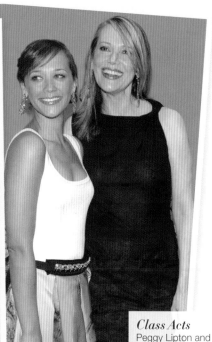

Class Acts
Peggy Lipton and
Rashida Jones prove
that a sweet, polished
streak is in the genes.

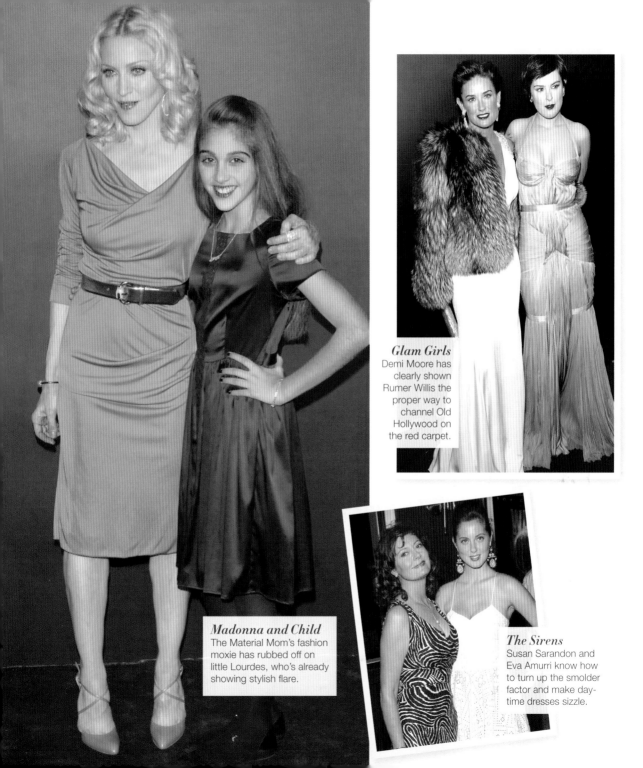

Glam Girls
Demi Moore has clearly shown Rumer Willis the proper way to channel Old Hollywood on the red carpet.

Madonna and Child
The Material Mom's fashion moxie has rubbed off on little Lourdes, who's already showing stylish flare.

The Sirens
Susan Sarandon and Eva Amurri know how to turn up the smolder factor and make daytime dresses sizzle.

PHOTO CREDITS

Cover: Patrick Demarchelier; Model: Carolyn Murphy.   Back Cover: Courtesy Dior.   Spine & Title Page: Davies + Starr.

Chapter 1 The Perfect Wardrobe

Page 8 Terry Tsiolis; Model: Liya Kebede. Page 10 Eric Ryan/Getty Images. Page 11 From left: PatrickMcMullan.com; Johnny Nunez/WireImage; PatrickMcMullan.com. Page 12 Vittorio Zunino Celotto/Getty Images. Page 13 From left: Eliot Press/Bauergriffinonline.com; PatrickMcMullan.com; Big Pictures/Bauergriffinonline.com. Page 14 From left: Jon Kopaloff/FilmMagic; Doug Meszler/Wenn; Gabriel Bouys/AFP/Getty Images. Page 16 Tim Rooke/Rex USA. Page 17 From left: Michael Loccisano/FilmMagic; JP Yim/WireImage; Michael Williams/Startraksphoto.com. Page 18 From left: Soul Brother/FilmMagic; Lester Cohen/WireImage. Page 19 From left: PatrickMcMullan.com; Bryan Bedder/Getty Images.

Chapter 2 Smart Shopping

Page 20 Greg Kadel; Model: Marina Linchuk. Page 22 From left: kika/x17online.com; Andrew H. Walker/Getty Images. Page 23 From left: David Fisher/Rex USA; Dan & Corina Lecca. Page 25 Anders Overgaard. Page 26 Still life: Davies + Starr. Page 27 Clockwise from top left: Richard Young/Startraksphoto.com (2); Humberto Carreno/Startraksphoto.com (2); James Devaney/WireImage; ZFI/Dave/ISBP/Danielle, Venturini, Olycom, and Venturini/All Bauergriffinonline.com. Page 28 Clockwise from top left: Pascal Le Segretain/Getty Images; PatrickMcMullan.com; Big Pictures/Bauergriffinonline.com; Radial Press/Startraksphoto.com. Still life: Davies + Starr; Courtesy Yves Saint Laurent. Page 29 Clockwise from top left: Dave M. Benett/Getty Images; Rex USA; Kazden/Rex USA; AFP/Getty Images; PRJ/Fame Pictures. Still life: Davies + Starr.

Chapter 3 How to Wear It: Tops

Page 30 Greg Kadel; Model: Anja Rubik; Page 32 Jean Baptiste Lacroix/WireImage. Page 33 From left: Michael Loccisano/FilmMagic; Broadimage; Jason Merritt/Getty Images. Pages 34-35 Dan & Corina Lecca. Still life: Davies + Starr; Nils Friedman/Studio D. Page 36 Tony Barson/WireImage. Page 37 From left: Ginsburg-Spaly/X17online.com; INFPhoto.com; Rex USA. Pages 38-39 Dan & Corina Lecca. Still life: Davies + Starr; Todd Huffman; Nils Friedman/Studio D; Courtesy Mawi. Page 40 Marion Curtis/Startraksphoto.com. Page 41 From left: Ray Tamarra/Getty Images; PatrickMcMullan.com; Andrew H. Walker/Getty Images. Pages 42-43 Dan & Corina Lecca; Still life: Jeffrey Westbrook/Studio D; Nils Friedman/Studio D; Davies + Starr; Todd Huffman. Page 44 From left: PatrickMcMullan.com; Michel DuFour; Dave Allocca/Startraksphoto.com. Page 45 Dan & Corina Lecca. Still life: Davies + Starr; Todd Huffman. Page 46 From left: Seth Browarnik/Startraksphoto.com; Paul Hawthorne/Startraksphoto.com; Stephanie Cardinale/People Avenue/Corbis; Jen Lowery/Startraksphoto.com. Page 47 Dan & Corina Lecca. Still life: Davies + Starr; Darryl Patterson.

Chapter 4 How to Wear It: Skirts

Page 48 Greg Kadel; Model: Arlenis Sosa. Page 50 Mike Marsland/WireImage. Page 51 From left: Dimitrios Kambouris/WireImage; Jean Baptiste Lacroix/WireImage; George Taylor/Everett/Rex USA. Pages 52-53 From left: Dan & Corina Lecca (2); Imaxtree; Dan & Corina Lecca; Imaxtree. Still life: Davies + Starr; Todd Huffman. Page 54 Beretta/Sims/Karius/Rex USA; Page 55 From left: Tony Barson/WireImage; Jamie McCarthy/WireImage; Charles Sykes/Rex USA. Pages 56-57 Imaxtree; Dan & Corina Lecca (4). Still life: Jeffrey Westbrook/Studio D; Nils Friedman/Studio D; Darryl Patterson; Davies + Starr; Courtesy Furla. Page 58 Splash News. Page 59 From left: PatrickMcMullan.com; Mike Coppola/FilmMagic; Michael Loccisano/Getty Images. Pages 60-61 From left: Dan & Corinna Lecca. Still life: Davies + Starr; Todd Huffman. Page 62 INFPhoto.com; Everett Collection/Rex USA; Bill Davila/Startraksphoto.com. Page 63 Clockwise from top left: Dan & Corina Lecca (2); Imaxtree. Still life: Davies + Starr. Page 64 From left: PatrickMcMullan.com; Jen Lowery/Startraksphoto.com; Stefanie Keenan/Getty Images; WWD/Conde Nast/Corbis. Page 65 From top: Dan & Corina Lecca; Imaxtree. Still life: Davies + Starr; Todd Huffman; Courtesy Christian Louboutin. Pages 66-67 Dan & Corina Lecca.

Chapter 5 How to Wear It: Jackets & Coats

Page 68 Greg Kadel; Model: Marina Linchuk. Pages 70 Revolutionpix/Bauergriffinonline.com. Page 71 From left Daniel/Cesar/INFPhoto.com; Michael Tran/FilmMagic; Michel DuFour. Pages 72-73 From left: Dan & Corina Lecca (3); Imaxtree. Still life: Davies + Starr; Darryl Patterson. Pages 74 Tony Barson/WireImage. Page 75 From left: Danielle Venturelli/WireImage; Sam Snap/FilmMagic; Barry Brecheisen/WireImage. Pages 76-77 From left: Imaxtree; Dan & Corina Lecca (2); Imaxtree. Still life: Davies + Starr; Darryl Patterson; Courtesy Tiffany & Co. Pages 78 Roger Wong/INFPhoto.com. Page 79 From left: Brian To/FilmMagic; Kika Press/X17online.com; ANG/Fame Pictures. Pages 80-81 From left: Dan & Corina Lecca (3); Kevin Sturman courtesy Prabal Gurung. Still life: Davies + Starr; Todd Huffman; Nils Friedman/Studio D; Courtesy Dolce & Gabbana. Pages 82 From left: Stephen Lovekin/Getty Images; Jim Spellman/WireImage; JM/X17online.com. Page 83 Dan & Corina Lecca. Still life: Davies + Starr; Nils Friedman/Studio D; Courtesy Marni. Pages 84 From left: Jamie McCarthy/WireImage; PatrickMcMullan.com; Mathew Imaging/WireImage; PatrickMcMullan.com. Page 85 Dan & Corina Lecca. Still life: Davies + Starr; Darryl Patterson; Courtesy Valextra; Courtesy H. Stern.

Chapter 6 How to Wear It: Pants

Page 86 Tom Munro; Model: Masha Novoselova; Pages 88 From left: PatrickMcMullan.com; Jen Lowery/Startraksphoto.com; INFPhoto.com. Page 89 Dan & Corina Lecca. Still life: Davies + Starr; Darryl Patterson; Courtesy Christian Louboutin. Pages 90 From left: Andy Fossum/Startraksphoto.com; Diane Cohen/Fame Pictures; Jim Spellman/WireImage. Page 91 Dan & Corina Lecca. Still life: Davies + Starr; Nils Friedman/Studio D; Darryl Patterson; Courtesy Mulberry. Page 92 From left: Nicolas Khayat/Enigma/Rex USA; Jennifer Livingston for Harper's Bazaar; Alberto E. Rodriguez/Getty Images. Page 93 Dan & Corina Lecca. Still life: Davies + Starr; Darryl Patterson; Todd Huffman. Page 94 From left: Paul Hawthorne/Startraksphoto.com; David Fisher/Rex USA; PatrickMcMullan.com. Page 95 Dan & Corina Lecca. Still life: Davies + Starr; Darryl Patterson. Page 96 From left: ANG/Fame Pictures; Astrid Stawiarz/Getty Images; Jackson Lee/Colin Drummond/Splashnews.com; PatrickMcMullan.com. Page 97 From top: Dan & Corina Lecca; Sean Cunningham. Still life: Davies + Starr; Darryl Patterson; Nils Friedman/Studio D; Courtesy Donna Karan; Courtesy Tiffany & Co. Pages 98-99 From left: Courtesy Devi Kroell (1); Dan & Corina Lecca.

Chapter 7 How to Wear It: Dresses

Page 100: Tom Munro; Model: Chanel Iman. Pages 102 Eamonn McCormack/WireImage. Page 103 From left Andrew H. Walker/Getty Images; PatrickMcMullan.com; INFPhoto.com. Pages 104-105 From left: Dan & Corina Lecca; Courtesy Doo Ri; Dan & Corina Lecca (2); Imaxtree. Still life: Davies + Starr; Todd Huffman; Darryl Patterson; Courtesy H. Stern. Pages 106 Nick Harvey/WireImage. Page 107 From left Marion Curtis/Startraksphoto.com; Vila/Anderson/Bauergriffinonline.com; Humberto Carreno/Startraksphoto.com. Pages 108-109 From left: Dan & Corina Lecca (4); Courtesy Devi Kroell. Still life: Davies + Starr; Nils Friedman/Studio D; Todd Huffman; Courtesy Cartier. Pages 110 From left: Michael N. Todaro/FilmMagic; Victor Chavez/WireImage; Pascal Le Segretain/Getty Images. Page 111 Dan & Corina Lecca; Still life: Davies + Starr; Jesus Ayala. Page 112 From left: Amanda Schwab/Startraksphoto.com; Andy Fossum/Startrakphotos.com; Nick Sadler/Startraksphoto.com; Page 113 Dan & Corina Lecca. Still life: Davies + Starr; Darryl Patterson. Page 114 From left: Roger Wong/INFPhoto.com; Fotonoticias/WireImage; Ferdaus Shamim/WireImage; Dominique Charriau/WireImage. Page 115 Dan & Corina Lecca. Still life: Davies + Starr; Darryl Patterson; Todd Huffman; Nils Friedman/Studio D.

Page 116 Greg Kadel; Model: Coco Rocha. Page 118 From left: Peter Brooker/Rex USA; Dave Allocca/Startraksphoto.com; Patrick McMullan.com. Page 119 Clockwise from top right: Imaxtree; Dan & Corina Lecca (2). Still life: Nils Friedman/Studio D; Davies + Starr. Page 120 From left: Kevin Mazur/Getty Images; PatrickMcMullan.com; Richard Young/Startraksphoto.com. Page 121 Dan & Corina Lecca; Still life: Davies + Starr. Page 122 From left: George Pimentel/WireImage; PatrickMcMullan. com; Mandel Ngan/AFP/Getty Images. Page 123 Clockwise from top right: Imaxtree; Dan & Corina Lecca (2). Still life: Davies + Starr; Darryl Patterson; Courtesy Pierre Hardy; Courtesy Louis Vuitton. Page 124 From left: Elizabeth Goodenough/Rex USA; Taylor Hill/FilmMagic; Rex USA; Page 125 Dan & Corina Lecca. Still life: Nils Friedman/Studio D; Davies + Starr; Courtesy Van Cleef & Arpels. Page 126 From left: Jemal Countess/WireImage; Jen Lowery/Startraksphoto.com; Jeff Kravitz/FilmMagic; PatrickMcMullan.com. Page 127 Dan & Corina Lecca. Still life: Davies + Starr; Darryl Patterson; Nils Friedman/Studio D; Courtesy Giorgio Armani; Courtesy Nina Ricci.

Chapter 9 Best Extras

Page 128 Greg Kadel; Model: Suvi Koponen.

Shoes

Page 130 Dimitrios Kambouris/WireImage. Page 131 Still life: Davies + Starr; Darryl Patterson; Todd Huffman; Courtesy Yves Saint Laurent. Courtesy Cesare Paciotti. Page 132 From left: Dan & Corina Lecca; Sean Cunningham; Dan & Corina Lecca. Still life: Darryl Patterson; Davies + Starr; Courtesy Stella McCartney. Page 133 From left: Eric Ryan/Getty Images; George Pimente/ WireImage; Humberto Carreno/Startraksphoto.com. Still life: Davies + Starr. Page 134 Picture Perfect/Rex USA. Page 135 Still life: Davies + Starr; Darryl Patterson; Nils Friedman/Studio D. Page 136 Clockwise from top left: Dan & Corina Lecca (4); Sean Cunningham. Still life: Davies + Starr. Page 137 From left: Jun Sato/WireImage; Eric Charbonneau/WireImage; James Devaney/ WireImage. Still life: Davies + Starr; Kevin Sweeney/Studio D; Courtesy Christian Louboutin. Page 138 PatrickMcMullan. com. Page 139 Still life: Davies + Starr; Darryl Patterson; Courtesy Pierre Hardy; Courtesy Dior; Courtesy Roger Vivier. Page 140 Clockwise from left: Dan & Corina Lecca; Sean Cunningham (2); Dan & Corina Lecca. Page 141 From left: Picture Perfect/ Rex USA; Rex USA; Stewart Cook/Rex USA. Still life: Davies + Starr; Nils Friedman/Studio D. Page 142 From left: Dominique Charriau/WireImage; Lorenzo Santini/WireImage. Still life: Nils Friedman/Studio D; Darryl Patterson. Page 143 From Clockwise from right: Dan & Corina Lecca; Sean Cunningham; Dan & Corina Lecca; Sean Cunningham (2). Still life: Davies + Starr. Page 144 From left: Dan & Corina Lecca; Sean Cunningham; Dave Allocca/Startraksphoto.com; Humberto Carreno/ Startraksphoto.com. Still life: Darryl Patterson; Davies + Starr; Todd Huffman. Page 145 From left: Pascal Le Segretain/Getty Images; Dave Allocca/Startraksphoto.com; Dan & Corina Lecca (2). Still life: Davies + Starr; Todd Huffman; Courtesy Christian Louboutin.

Bags

Page 146 Vila/Krieger/Bauergriffinonline.com. Page 147 Still life: Davies + Starr; Todd Huffman; Darryl Patterson; Chris Eckerts/Studio D; Courtesy Smythson and Gerard Yosca; Courtesy Anya Hindmarch; Courtesy Dior. Page 148 Clockwise from top left: Sean Cunningham (2); Dan & Corina Lecca; Sean Cunningham; Dan & Corina Lecca. Still life: Davies + Starr; Courtesy Etro. Page 149 From left: PatrickMcMullan.com (2); Fame Pictures. Still life: Todd Huffman; Nils Friedman/Studio D; Courtesy Mulberry. Page 150 Kevin Mazur/WireImage. Page 151 Still life: Davies + Starr; Todd Huffman; Darryl Patterson; Courtesy Goyard; Courtesy Prada. Page 152 Clockwise from top left: Sean Cunningham; Dan & Corina Lecca (4); Still life: Davies + Starr. Page 153 From left: Jen Lowery/Startraksphoto.com; Andrew H. Walker/Getty Images; Beretta Sims/Rex USA. Still life: Davies + Starr; Todd Huffman. Page 154 PatrickMcMullan.com; Page 155 Still life: Davies + Starr; Todd Huffman; Darryl Patterson; Chris Eckert/Studio D. Page 156 Clockwise from left: Sean Cunningham; Dan & Corina Lecca (4); Still life: Davies + Starr; Courtesy Marni. Page 157 From left: Eric Feferberg/AFP/Getty Images; PatrickMcMullan.com; Humberto Carreno/Startraksphoto. com. Still life: Davies + Starr; Darryl Patterson. Pate 158 From left: Michel Dufour; Patrick McMullan.com. Still life: Davies + Starr. Page 159 Clockwise from top left: Sean Cunningham; Dan & Corina Lecca (2); Sean Cunningham (2). Still life: Davies

+ Starr. Page 160 From left: PatrickMcMullan.com; Dominique Charriau/WireImage; Sean Cunningham; Courtesy Marni. Still life: Davies + Starr; Todd Huffman; Darryl Patterson; Kevin Sweeney/Studio D. Page 161 From left: Dan & Corina Lecca; Sean Cunningham; Steven Hirsch/Splash News; PatrickMcMullan.com. Still life: Davies + Starr; Courtesy Valentino; Courtesy Salvatore Ferragamo.

Scarves

Page 162 From left: Humberto Carreno/Startraksphoto.com; Goff/INFphoto.com; Big Pictures/Bauergriffinonline.com. Page 163 From left: Charley Gallay/WireImage; PatrickMcMullan.com (2). Still life: Nils Friedman/Studio D; Phyllis Baker/Studio D; Jesus Ayala/Studio D; Davies + Starr.

Belts

Page 164 From left: Michael Williams/Startraksphoto.com; PatrickMcMullan.com; Peter Kramer/Getty Images. Page 165 From left: Rex USA; Jordan Strauss/WireImage; Dan Herrick/KPA/Zuma Press. Still life: Davies + Starr.

Jewelry

Page 166 From left: Jen Lowery/Startraksphoto.com; Frederick M. Brown/Getty Images; Sean Cunningham; Dan & Corina Lecca. Still life: Davies + Starr; Darryl Patterson. Page 167 From left: Dan & Corina Lecca (2); Gustavo Caballero/WireImage; Axelle/Bauergriffinonline.com. Still life: Davies + Starr; Darryl Patterson; David Kressler/Courtesy Dean Harris. Page 168 From left: Jeff Vespa/WireImage; Jen Lowery/Startraksphoto.com; Dan & Corina Lecca; Simon Burstall. Still life: Nils Friedman/Studio D; Todd Huffman; Davies + Starr; Chris Eckert/Studio D. Page 169 From left: Dan & Corina Lecca (2); Jim Spellman/WireImage; Erik C. Pendzich/Rex USA. Still life: Davies + Starr; Jesus Ayala/Studio D; Jeffrey Westbrook/Studio D. Page 170 From left: Eric Ryan/Getty Images; Rex USA; Sean Cunningham; Dan & Corina Lecca. Still life: Davies + Starr; Courtesy Montblanc; Courtesy Cartier; Courtesy Rolex. Page 171 From left: Dan & Corina Lecca (2); PatrickMcMullan.com; Visual/Zuma Press. Still life: Davies + Starr; Courtesy Breil Milano; Courtesy Harry Winston.

Chapter 10 Beach Guide

Page 172 Alexi Lubomirski; Model: Karmen Pedaru. Page 174 From left: Dan & Corina Lecca; John Calabrese/Gaz Shirley/PacificCoastNews.com; Dan & Corina Lecca. Still life: Davies + Starr; Todd Huffman; Courtesy Ray-Ban. Page 175 From left: Sean Cunningham; Eliot Press/Bauergriffinonline.com; Dan & Corina Lecca. Still life: Davies + Starr. Page 176 From left: Ben McDonald/Bauergriffinonline.com; Sean Cunningham; Dan & Corina Lecca. Still life: Davies + Starr; Todd Huffman. Page 177 From left: Sean Cunningham; Everett Collection/Rex USA; Dan & Corina Lecca. Still life: Davies + Starr; Todd Huffman. Page 178 From left: Flynet; Dan & Corina Lecca (2). Still life: Davies + Starr; Nils Friedman/Studio D; Courtesy Karl Lagerfeld. Page 179 From left: ©StefanoGuindaniPhoto; Dan & Corina Lecca (2). Still life: Davies + Starr; Todd Huffman; Darryl Patterson.

The Last Word

Page 182 Clockwise from top right: Eliot Press/Bauergriffinonline.com; PatrickMcMullan.com (2). Page 183 Clockwise from left: PatrickMcMullan.com; Neilson Barnard/Getty Images; PatrickMcMullan.com.

Library of Congress Cataloging-in-Publication Data
D'Souza, Nandini.
 Harper's Bazaar fabulous at every age / by Nandini D'Souza ; edited by Jenny Barnett.
    p. cm.
 Includes index.
 ISBN 978-1-58816-809-2
 1. Fashion. 2. Women's clothing. I. Barnett, Jenny. II. Harper's Bazaar. III. Title.
 TT507.D735 2009
 746.9'2--dc22
                    2009016689

Published by Hearst Books
A division of Sterling Publishing Co., Inc.
387 Park Avenue South, New York, NY 10016

Harper's Bazaar and Hearst Books are trademarks of Hearst Communications, Inc.

www.harpersbazaar.com

Writer: Nandini D'Souza
Editor: Jenny Barnett
Production: Tom McKee
Photo Editor: Georgia Paralemos
Digital Imaging Specialist: Erica Parente
Designer: Bess Yoham
With thanks to: Ashley Curry, Jil Derryberry, Elizabeth Hummer, Karin Kato, Lisa M. Luna,
Victoria Pedersen, Melanie M. Ryan, Sarah Strzelec, Amber Vanderzee

For information about custom editions, special sales, premium, and corporate purchases, please contact
Sterling Special Sales Department at 800-805-5489 or specialsales@sterlingpublishing.com.

Distributed in Canada by Sterling Publishing
c/o Canadian Manda Group, 165 Dufferin Street
Toronto, Ontario, Canada M6K 3H6

Distributed in Australia by Capricorn Link (Australia) Pty. Ltd.
P.O. Box 704, Windsor, NSW 2756 Australia

Distributed in the United Kingdom by GMC Distribution Services
Castle Place, 166 High Street, Lewes, East Sussex, England BN7 1XU

Manufactured in China

Sterling ISBN 978-1-58816-809-2